STATISTICS IN PRACTICE

An Illustrated Guide to SPSS

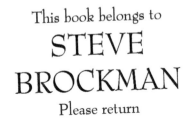

This book belongs to
STEVE
BROCKMAN
Please return

STATISTICS IN PRACTICE

An Illustrated Guide to SPSS

Basant K Puri

MA MB MChir MRCPsych

Senior Research Fellow, Robert Steiner Magnetic Resonance Unit,
Royal Postgraduate Medical School, Hammersmith Hospital, London, UK

A member of the Hodder Headline Group
LONDON • SYDNEY • AUCKLAND
Co-published in the USA by Oxford University Press, Inc., New York

First published in Great Britain 1996 by
Arnold, a member of the Hodder Headline Group,
338 Euston Road, London NW1 3BH

Co-published in the United States of America by
Oxford University Press Inc.,
198 Madison Avenue, New York, NY 10016
Oxford is a registered trademark of Oxford University Press

British Library Cataloguing in Publication Data
A catalogue record for this book is available from the British Library

Library of Congress Cataloging-in-Publication Data
A catalog record for this book is available from the Library of Congress

ISBN 0 340 66209 3

Typeset in 9/11 pt Palatino by GreenGate Publishing Services, Tonbridge, Kent
Printed and bound in Great Britain by J. W. Arrowsmith, Bristol

CONTENTS

PREFACE

This book offers a practical guide to using SPSS for Windows. Details are given of how to choose, access and use a variety of statistical procedures and charts available in this powerful statistics package. Rather than doing this by giving lists of commands, screen shots have been used that correspond to what the user actually sees on the computer monitor.

I should like to thank SPSS for giving me permission to reproduce screen shots from their software.

Basant K Puri,
Cambridge, England

PREFACE

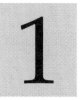

INTRODUCTION

AIMS OF THIS BOOK

This book provides a practical guide to using a popular statistical software package, SPSS for Windows. The screen shots in the book are taken from version 6.1 of the software.

The book considers the following aspects of the use of SPSS:

- data entry
- the choice of an appropriate statistical test
- exploring the data
- data transformation
- running statistical tests and producing graphical (chart) images.

In general, details of the theory underlying the statistical tests described are not provided; these are available in standard textbooks. Therefore mathematical formulae and equations have been omitted.

BASIC CONCEPTS

Variables

DEFINITION

A variable is an observable quantity or attribute that varies from one member of the population being studied to another.

CLASSIFICATION

Figure 1.1 shows one way in which variables can be classified.

INDEPENDENT AND DEPENDENT VARIABLES

The variable whose values you wish to predict or summarize is the dependent variable, while the variable(s) it depends on is (are) the independent variable(s).

Measurement scales

There are four main types of measurement scale that can be used for different types of data: nominal, ordinal, interval and ratio. Their characteristics are summarized in Table 1.1.

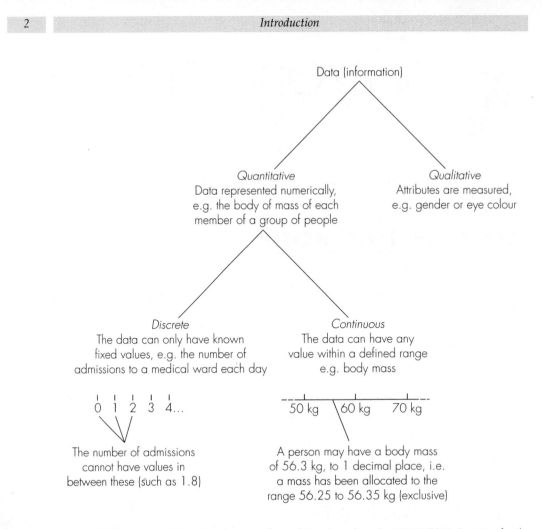

Figure 1.1 Summary of the classification of variables. Based on Puri BK (1996) *Statistics for the Health Sciences*, with permission from WB Saunders, London

TABLE 1.1 Types of measurement scale. Based on Puri BK (1996) *Statistics for the Health Sciences*, with permission from WB Saunders, London

Property	Nominal	Ordinal	Interval	Ratio
Categories mutually exclusive	✓	✓	✓	✓
Categories logically ordered		✓	✓	✓
Equal distance between adjacent categories			✓	✓
True zero point				✓

NOMINAL

A nominal measurement scale is a set of mutually exclusive categories that varies qualitatively but not quantitatively, for example gender and eye colour. For computational purposes, numbers are attached to these categories when using SPSS, but these numbers do not imply that any one category is higher than another. For instance, when measuring eye colour, 1 may stand for blue, 2 for brown, 3 for green, and so on, but this does not imply that the categories are unequal.

ORDINAL

An ordinal measurement scale differs from a nominal one in that the order among the original categories is preserved in the analysis; however, differences between adjacent categories are not equal. Examples include social class and the staging of cancer. Numbers attached to these categories reflect their relative order. For example, social class 1 is higher than social class 3; however, the difference between social classes 1 and 3 is not the same as the difference between social classes 3 and 5 (even though numerically $3 - 1 = 5 - 3$). In other words the numbers just give the rank.

The ordinal scale is more informative than the nominal scale. Variables measured on nominal and ordinal scales are discrete variables.

INTERVAL

An interval scale differs from an ordinal one in that the differences between adjacent categories are equal; however, there is no true zero point. Examples include the Fahrenheit and Celsius temperature scales. For example, 60°C is a higher temperature than 50°C, and the difference in temperature between 60°C and 50°C is the same as the difference between 30°C and 20°C; however, 60°C is not twice the temperature of 30°C, since 0°C is not absolute zero.

The interval scale is more informative than nominal and ordinal scales.

RATIO

A ratio scale differs from an interval one in that there is a true zero point. Examples include the measurement of height in metres and the Kelvin temperature scale. For example, not only is the difference in height between 0.5 m and 0.4 m the same as the difference between 0.25 m and 0.15 m, but 0.5 m is twice 0.25 m.

The ratio scale is more informative than the preceding three scales. When using SPSS, it is usually sufficient to class variables measured on both interval and ratio scales together as continuous variables.

Parametric and nonparametric tests

Parametric tests (such as the *t*-test and analysis of variance (ANOVA)) make a number of assumptions about the data being analyzed:

- the dependent variable is continuous (that is, it is measured on an interval or ratio scale)
- the underlying population from which the sample data are taken has a normal distribution
- when differences or measures of statistical association are being analyzed between two or more samples, the variances (or standard deviations) of these samples do not differ significantly.

On the other hand, nonparametric tests (such as the chi-square test and the Mann–Whitney U test) do not make such assumptions.

If continuous data do not fulfil the assumptions of a parametric test, they can be converted into ordinal data and a nonparametric equivalent test can be used instead. However, in such a conversion, useful information is discarded from the data. It should also be borne in mind that most parametric tests are usually robust to small deviations from the strict criteria outlined above.

If the assumptions of a parametric test *are* fulfilled, then conversion of continuous data into ordinal data and using a nonparametric test result in a loss of statistical power. (The power of a hypothesis test is the probability that the null hypothesis is rejected when it is indeed false.)

USING MICROSOFT WINDOWS

It is assumed that the reader is familiar with the use of the Microsoft Windows environment. If not, then it is strongly recommended that the on-line tutorial available in Windows should be worked through. In Windows 3.1 and Windows for Workgroups 3.11 this is available from the Help menu of the Program Manager, as shown in Figure 1.2.

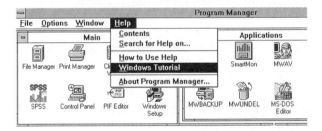

Figure 1.2 Accessing the Windows tutorial in Windows version 3.1/Windows for Workgroups version 3.11

USING SPSS FOR WINDOWS

If the reader has not previously used SPSS, then it is recommended that the SPSS tutorial should be worked through first. This is accessed as shown in Figure 1.3. The resulting main menu is shown in Figure 1.4.

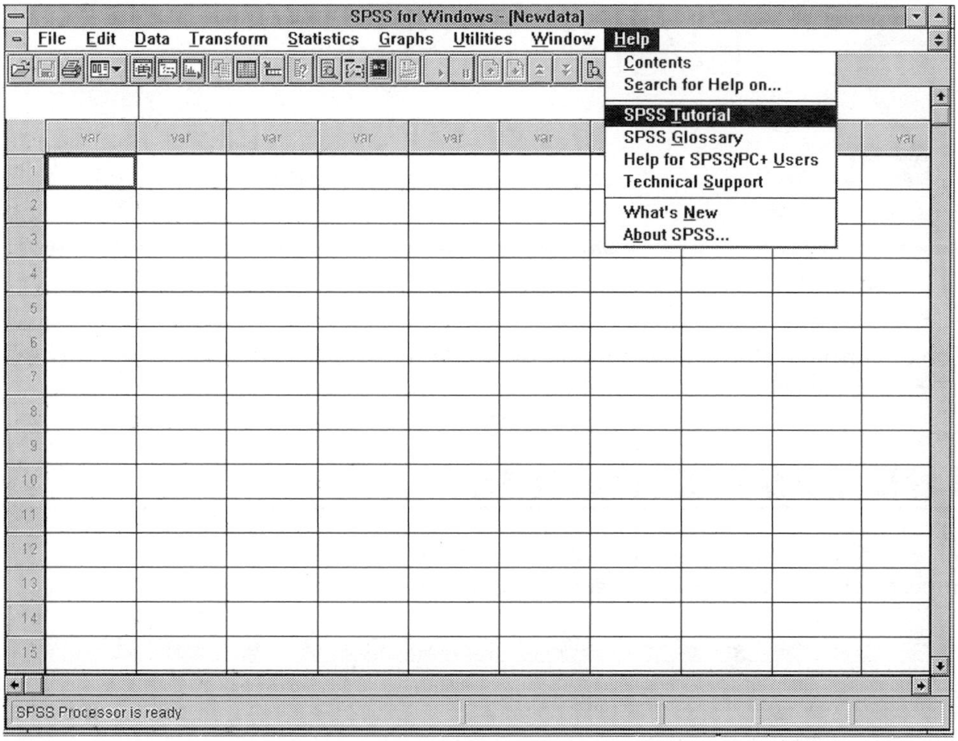

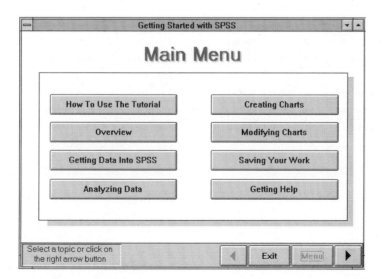

Figure 1.3 Accessing the SPSS tutorial in SPSS for Windows version 6.1

Figure 1.4 Main menu of the SPSS tutorial

2 DATA ENTRY

The data from a study, that is the information to be analyzed, are entered into an SPSS data file using the Data Editor.

THE SPSS DATA FILE

An example of a data file is shown in Figure 2.1.
Superficially, the Data Editor resembles a spreadsheet.

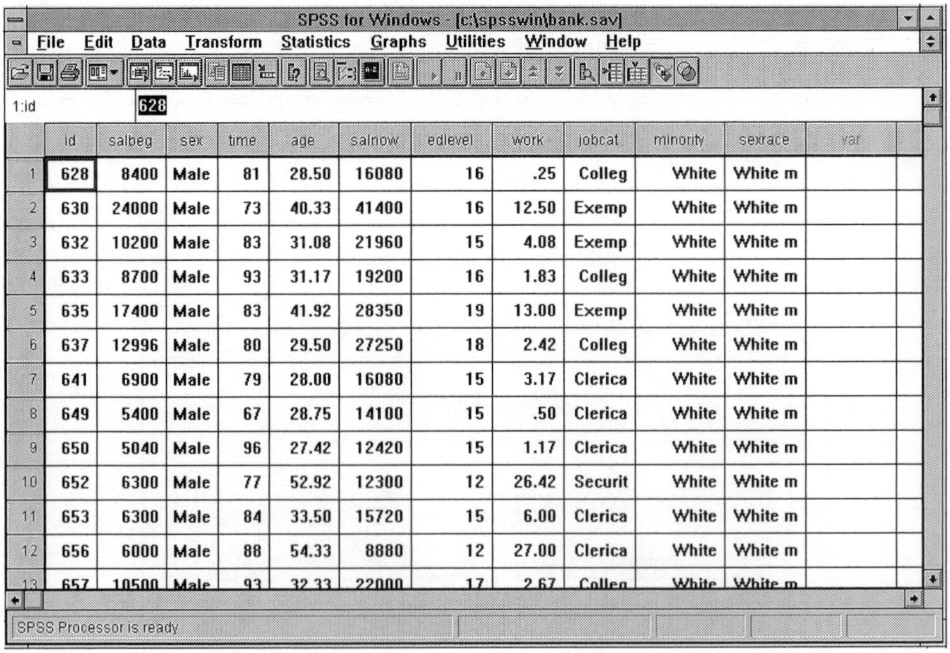

Figure 2.1 An example of a data file (taken from the sample data file bank.sav provided with SPSS)

Rows

Each row in the data file represents a single case. In Figure 2.2, for example, the highlighted row represents a person with identification (id) number 630. From this row it can be seen that this person is a white male who, at the time of data collection, was aged 40.33 years with a salary of $41 400, and so on.

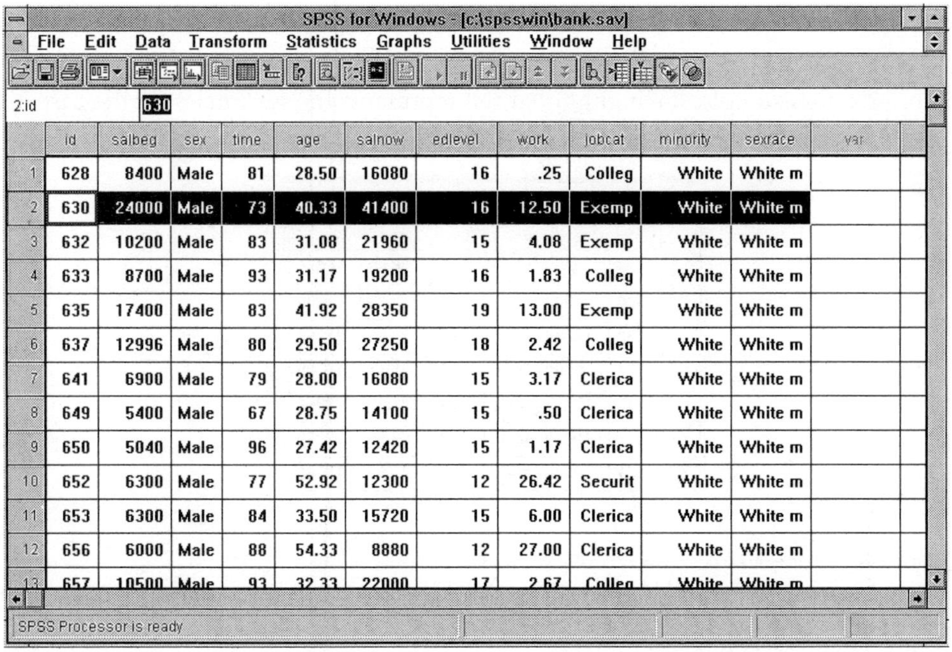

Figure 2.2 A single case is represented by a row

Columns

Each column represents a single variable. In Figure 2.3, for example, the highlighted column represents the sex of the individuals.

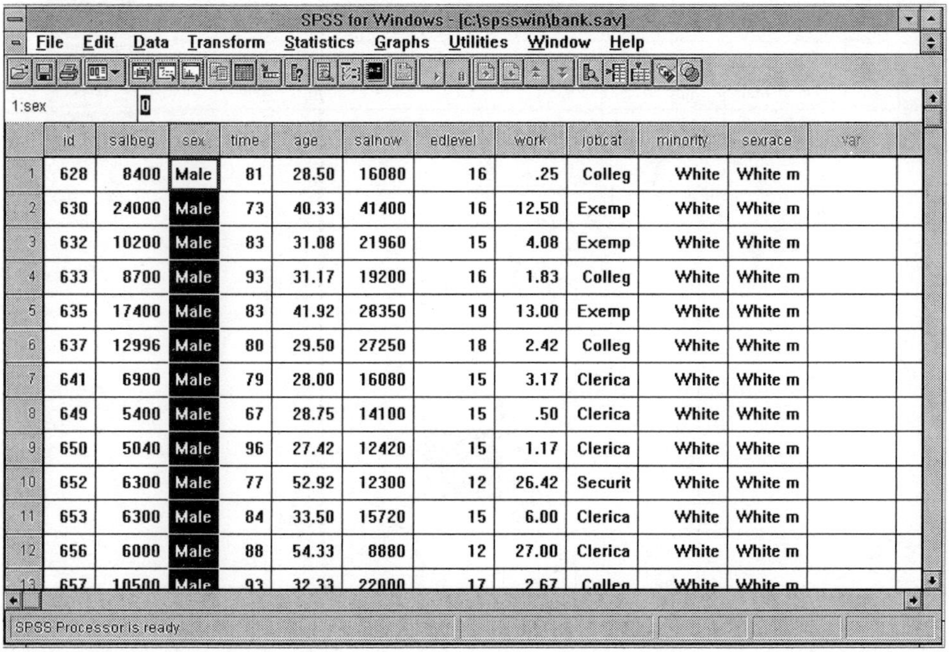

Figure 2.3 A single variable is represented by a column

Cells

The value of each cell is determined by its row (case) and column (variable). In Figure 2.4, for example, the highlighted cell represents the sex (male) for the case in row number one (the person with id 628).

	id	salbeg	sex	time	age	salnow
1	628	8400	Male	81	28.50	16080
2	630	24000	Male	73	40.33	41400
3	632	10200	Male	83	31.08	21960
4	633	8700	Male	93	31.17	19200
5	635	17400	Male	83	41.92	28350
6	637	12996	Male	80	29.50	27250
7	641	6900	Male	79	28.00	16080

1:sex   0

Figure 2.4 The value of a cell is determined by its row and column

Cells contain a period/full stop when they are empty (Figure 2.5) or when they correspond to missing data (Figure 2.6).

1:var00001

	id	salbeg	sex	time	age	salnow	edlevel	work	jobcat	minority	sexrace	var00001
1	628	8400	Male	81	28.50	16080	16	.25	Colleg	White	White m	.
2	630	24000	Male	73	40.33	41400	16	12.50	Exemp	White	White m	.
3	632	10200	Male	83	31.08	21960	15	4.08	Exemp	White	White m	.
4	633	8700	Male	93	31.17	19200	16	1.83	Colleg	White	White m	.
5	635	17400	Male	83	41.92	28350	19	13.00	Exemp	White	White m	.
6	637	12996	Male	80	29.50	27250	18	2.42	Colleg	White	White m	.

Figure 2.5 Empty cells (highlighted)

78	32.92	29400	19	3.75	Colleg
97	31.92	10920	12	5.50	Clerica
96	39.33	24150	19	8.00	Colleg
94	36.00	13920	15	7.75	Office t
78	63.75	12300	.	35.75	Securit
83	38.42	11736	.	12.50	Clerica
96	30.33	13020	.	3.58	Office t
95	33.75	14040	15	7.50	Clerica
78	35.42	16020	15	11.08	Exemp
98	35.67	16080	16	3.00	Clerica

Figure 2.6 Cells with missing data cells (highlighted)

THE DATA EDITOR

Data are entered into a data file using the data editor.

STANDARD NUMERICAL DATA

In SPSS, a numeric (numerical) variable refers to a variable whose values are displayed in standard numerical format, using the decimal point delimiter specified in the International Control Panel of the Program Manager of Windows; for example 0.37. As well as accepting numerical data in this standard format, data can be entered using scientific notation (see Figure 2.13 below) in which, for instance, $3.7E-1 = 3.7 \times 10^{-1} = 0.37$. The SPSS default is to accept numerical data in standard format during data entry.

Numerical data are entered by selecting the appropriate cells (using the mouse or cursor keys) and typing in the required numbers. Each value appears in the cell editor (Figure 2.7), where it can be edited, if necessary, before it is entered.

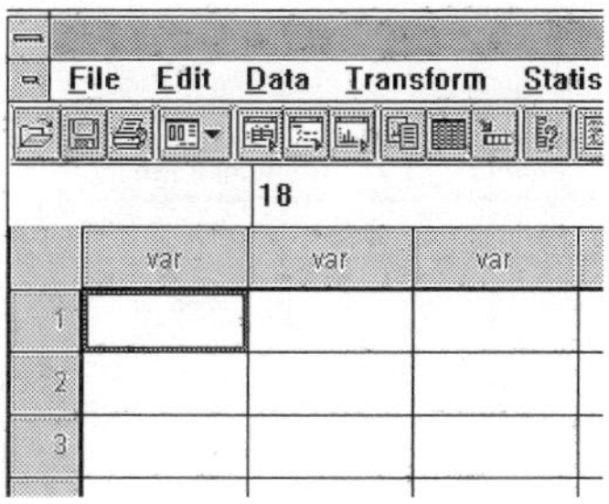

Figure 2.7 The cell editor

After **Enter** (or a cursor key) is pressedthe data value is entered into the data file, as shown in Figure 2.8. Note that if you have not defined the name of the variable, then SPSS gives it a unique name (in this case var00001). How to define a variable name is described in the next section.

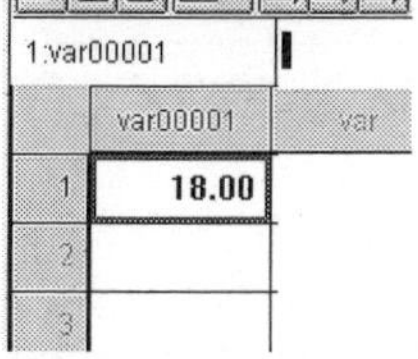

Figure 2.8 Entered data value with a default SPSS variable name

OTHER TYPES OF DATA

Defining variables

To enter other types of data, first the variable must be defined. The Define Variable box can be opened in SPSS for Windows version 6.1 simply by double clicking (with the left mouse button) the variable name at the head of the column, as shown in Figure 2.9.

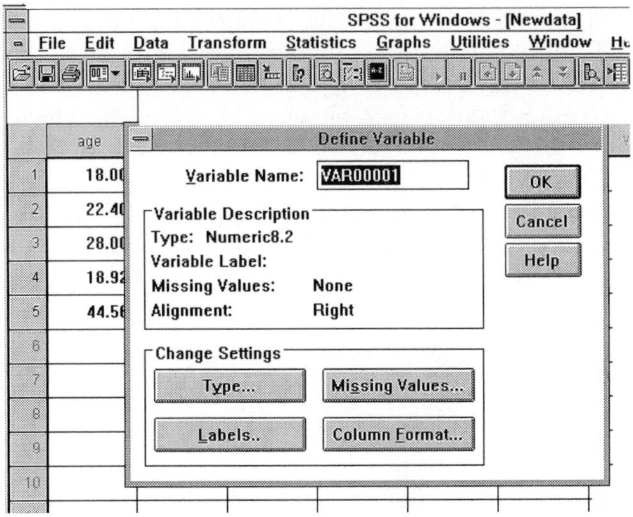

Figure 2.9 The Define Variable box

The variable name is highlighted and can be altered to the name of your choice (Figure 2.10).

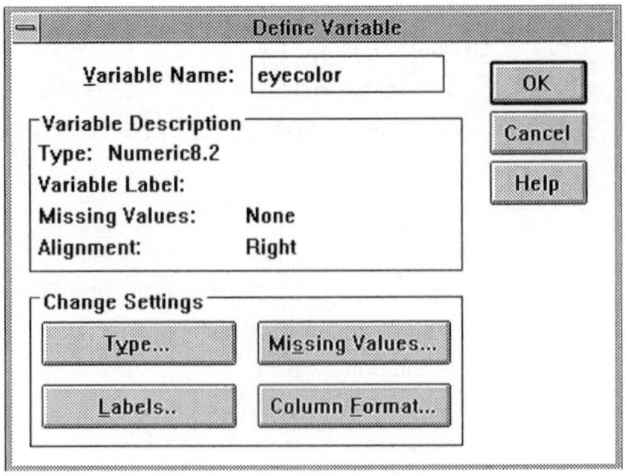

Figure 2.10 Defining a variable name

Alternatively, the Define Variable box can be opened using the Data menu (by means of the mouse or keyboard), as shown in Figure 2.11; this method must also be used with some older versions of SPSS.

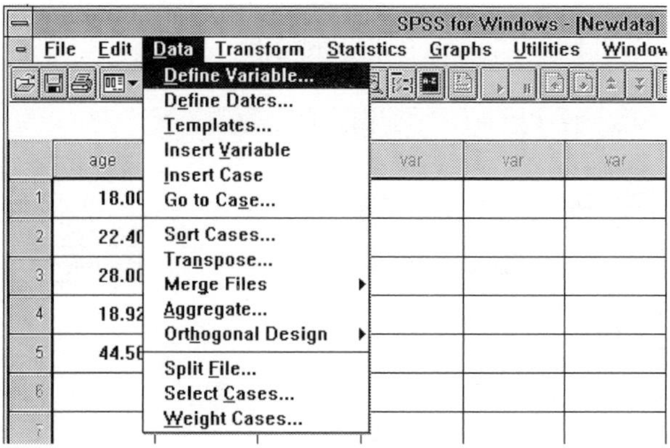

Figure 2.11 An alternative way of opening the **Define Variable** box

In the Define Variable box (see Figures 2.9 and 2.10) click on the Type... button. This opens the Define Variable Type box shown in Figure 2.12.

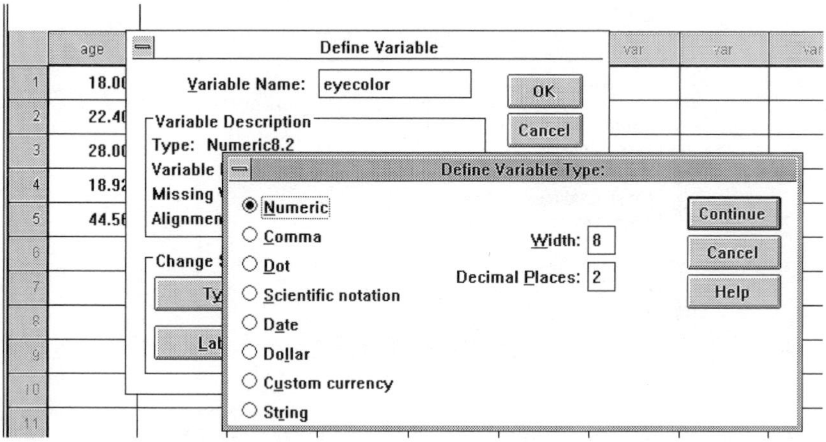

Figure 2.12 The **Define Variable Type** box

SPSS allows the entry of the following types of data:

● numeric – numerical data in standard format (see above)
● comma – a numerical variable with values displayed with commas dividing every three places, and with a period as a decimal delimiter
● dot – a numerical variable with values displayed with periods dividing every three places, and with a comma as a decimal delimiter
● scientific notation - see above
● date – a number of formats are available for displaying dates (for example when entering dates of birth)
● dollar
● custom currency
● string – the values can contain any characters up to the length defined in the Define Variable Type box; upper and lower case letters are considered to be different.

Suppose we want to choose a string variable with eight characters; then the Define Variable Type box will be as shown in Figure 2.13.

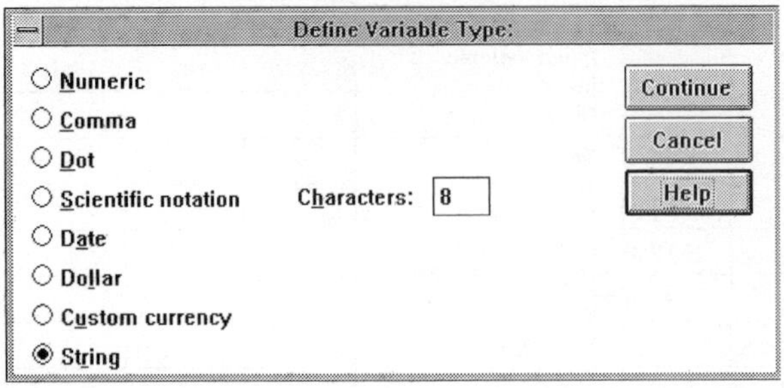

Figure 2.13 Choosing a variable type

Press on the Continue button. This leads to the altered Define Variable box shown in Figure 2.14, in which the variable is now defined as a string variable with up to eight characters (String8).

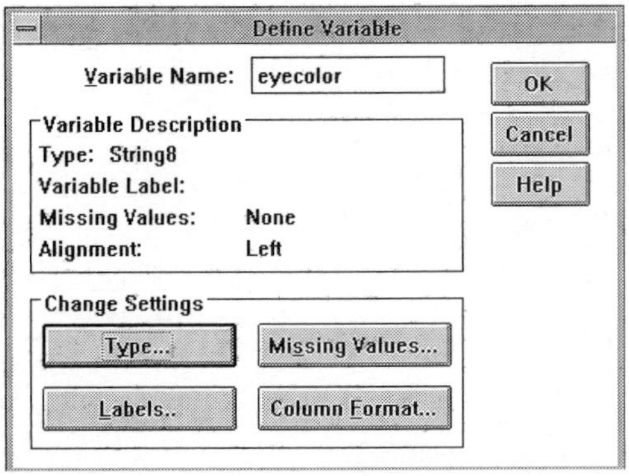

Figure 2.14 Define Variable box in which the variable is defined as a string variable with up to eight characters

Clicking on the OK button then results in the altered data file shown in Figure 2.15.

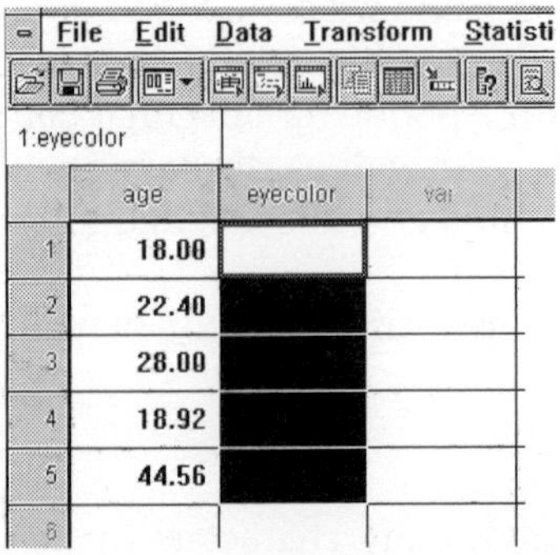

Figure 2.15 Altered data file with the new variable labelled eyecolor

Value labels

The string data for this new variable (eyecolor) could now be entered manually, word by word. However, an easier way of doing this is to define labels for these non-numerical data values. To do this, open the Define Variable box (for example by double clicking the variable name at the head of the column) and this time click on Labels... . This results in the Define Labels box shown in Figure 2.16.

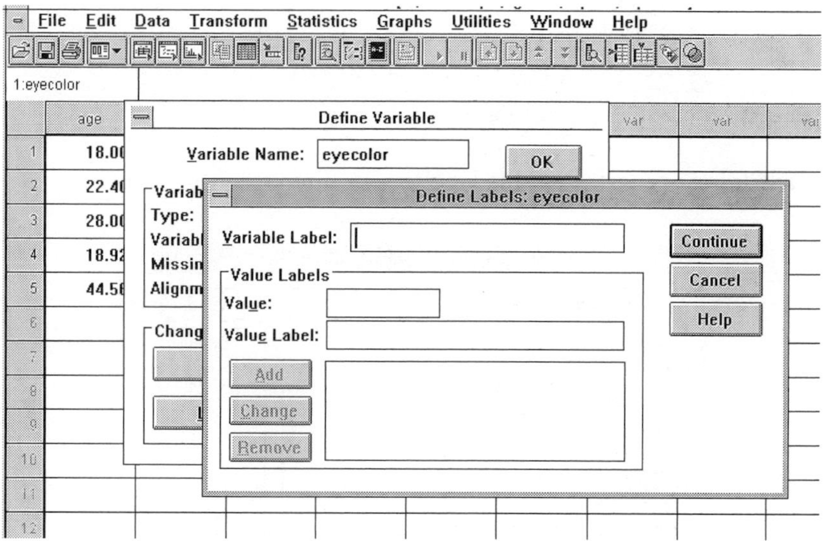

Figure 2.16 The Define Labels box

Fill in the full name of the variable label. We shall assign the number 1 to the eye colour blue by completing the box as shown in Figure 2.17.

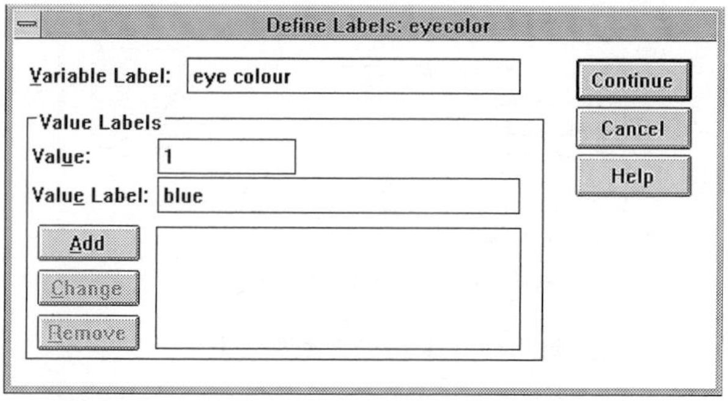

Figure 2.17 Filling in the Define Labels box

Then click on the Add button; this gives the result shown in Figure 2.18.

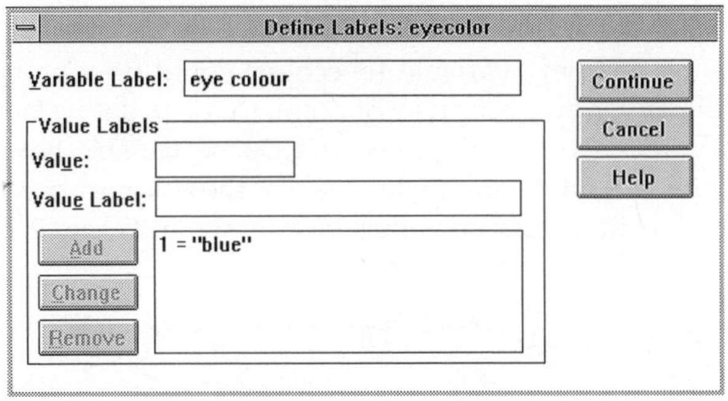

Figure 2.18 The result of clicking on **Add**

Continue adding as many variable labels as required (Figure 2.19).

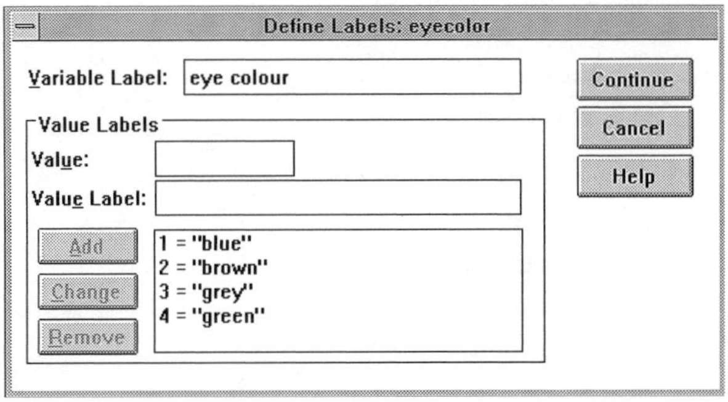

Figure 2.19 A complete list of variable labels

When all the variable labels have been added, click the **Continue** button. You then return to the **Define Variable** box, in which the full variable label now appears (Figure 2.20). If at any time more labels need to be added, or existing ones edited, this can be done simply by repeating the above process.

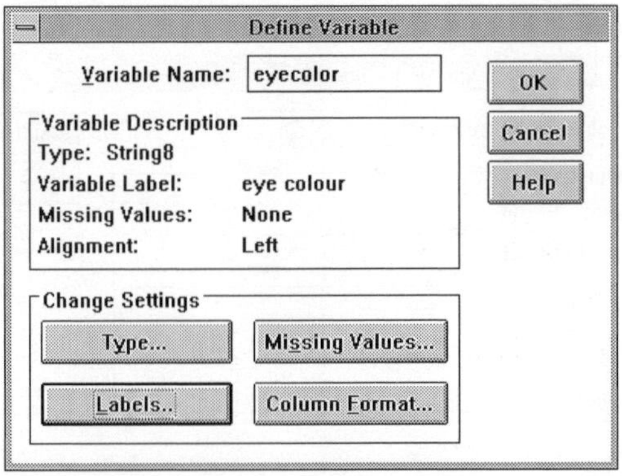

Figure 2.20 Modified **Define Variable** box with variable label now inserted

Click on OK in the **Define Variable** box and return to the data file. You can now enter data in the corresponding variable column simply by typing in the numbers corresponding to the labels you require (for example, 1 for blue, and so on). However, this means you have to remember the labelling, and this can become difficult as the number of non-numerical variables that you have labelled increases. To circumvent this difficulty, you can simply place the cursor in the required cell and click on the right mouse button to bring up a list of labels for that variable (Figure 2.21). You can then double click the left mouse button to choose the appropriate label.

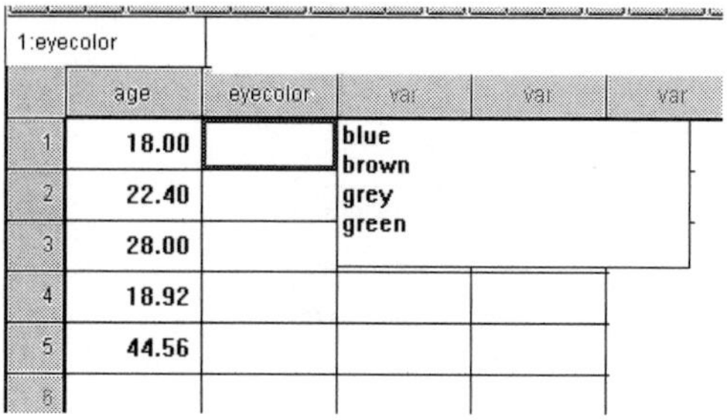

Figure 2.21 Displaying the list of labels for a non-numerical variable using the right mouse button

The filled-in variable column can simply display the label numbers as shown in Figure 2.22.

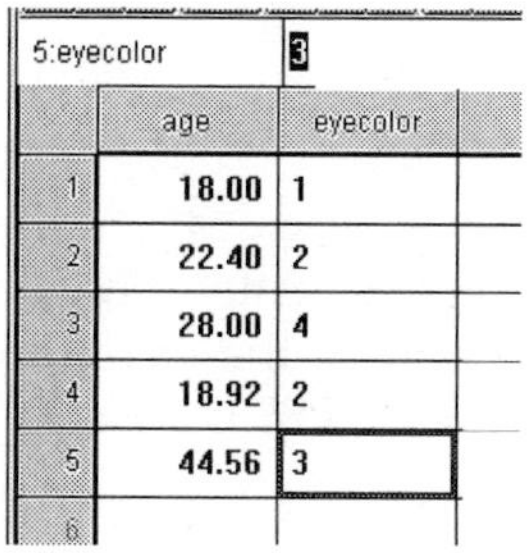

Figure 2.22 The label numbers displayed for the variable eyecolor

It is often more convenient, however, to display the actual value labels. This is done by selecting Value Labels from Utilities, as shown in Figure 2.23.

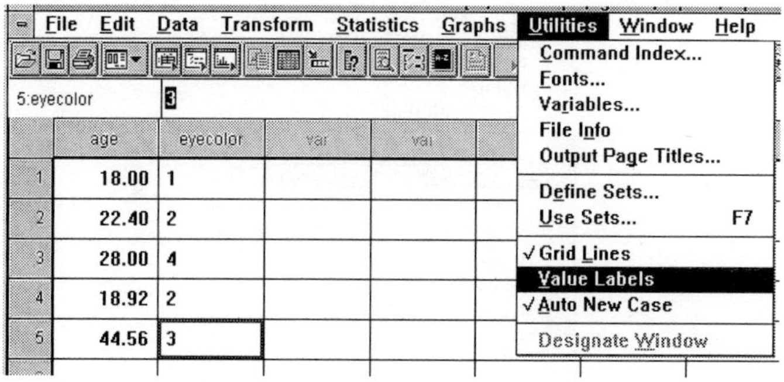

Figure 2.23 Selecting Value Labels from Utilities

Alternatively, the Value Labels button on the toolbar (Figure 2.24) can be clicked.

Figure 2.24 The **Value Labels** button on the toolbar

As a result, the value labels are now displayed in the data file (Figure 2.25).

5:eyecolor		
	age	eyecolor
1	18.00	blue
2	22.40	brown
3	28.00	green
4	18.92	brown
5	44.56	grey

Figure 2.25 The value labels displayed for the variable eyecolor

Without giving strings (such as eye colours) numerical value labels when entering them into the data file, you would limit the number of statistical operations SPSS could perform on these data.

Contingency tables

Thus far we have looked at how to enter raw data from actual observations. Sometimes, however, summary data in the form of contingency tables need to be entered. The way to carry this out in SPSS is described in Chapter 7.

Saving data

To save your new data file, select **Save Data** from the **File** menu, if you have made changes to a pre-existing data file, or select **Save As...** if you are saving a new data file or wish to save the changes in a new file (Figure 2.26).

```
File   Edit   Data   Transform   Statist
New                          ▶
Open                         ▶
Read ASCII Data...

Close
Save Data
Save As...
Export Chart...

Display Data Info...
Apply Data Dictionary...
Apply Chart Template...

Print...
Printer Setup...
Stop SPSS Processor    F3

Exit
```

Figure 2.26 Saving a data file

Alternatively, you can click the Save button on the toolbar (Figure 2.27).

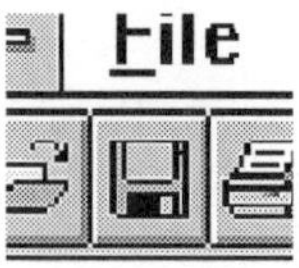

Figure 2.27 The Save button on the toolbar

OPENING A DATA FILE

To open a pre-existing data file, either use the File menu, as shown in Figure 2.28, or click the Open File button on the toolbar (Figure 2.29).

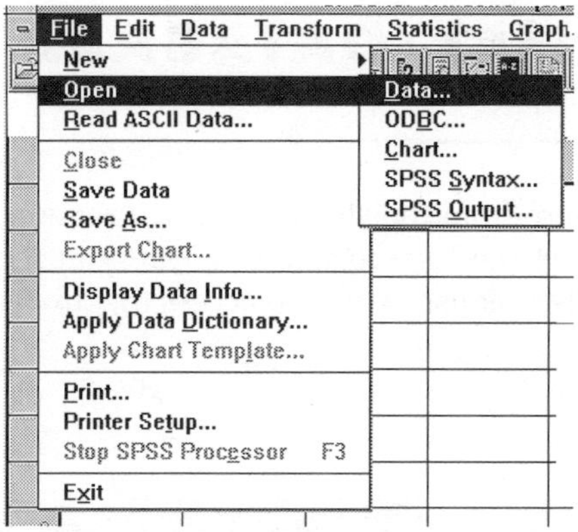

Figure 2.28 Opening a data file using the File menu

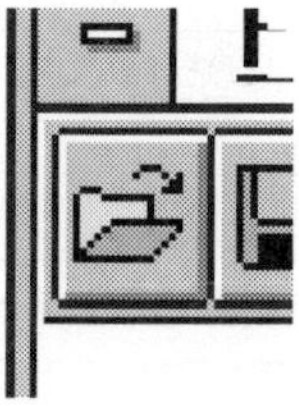

Figure 2.29 The Open File button on the toolbar

This opens the Open Data File box, from which the appropriate data file can be chosen in the usual way (Figure 2.30).

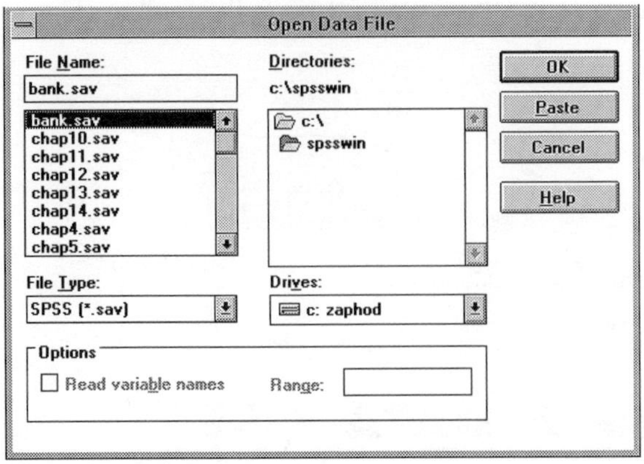

Figure 2.30 The Open Data File box

READING A SPREADSHEET/DATABASE INTO SPSS

The main difference here from the steps in the last section is that in the Open Data File box you must select the appropriate File Type you require, by clicking on the down arrow with the left mouse button to access the drop-down menu as shown in Figure 2.31.

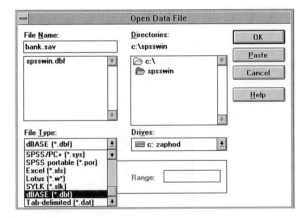

Figure 2.31 Choosing the appropriate File Type

If you have imported a spreadsheet, then its first row will probably contain the variable names, which you must then read into the SPSS data file by clicking on Read Variable Names in the Options group of the Open Data File box (Figure 2.32).

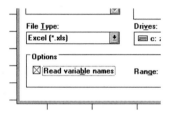

Figure 2.32 Reading column headings of a spreadsheet into SPSS data file variable names

If there are initial empty rows and/or columns in the spreadsheet, then you must let the SPSS program know the range of cells from which you want to read by entering this in the Range box of the Options group of the Open Data File box. The same format as is used for spreadsheets should be used here. For example, the cells in the rectangle with corners B3 and G10, inclusive, would be entered as B3:G10 (Figure 2.33).

File Type: **Drives:**

| Excel (*.xls) ± | | 🖳 c: zaphod ± |

Options

⊠ Read variable names   **Range:** `B3:G10`

Figure 2.33 Entering the spreadsheet range of cells to be read from

READING AN ASCII TEXT DATA FILE INTO SPSS

First select Read ASCII Data... from the File menu (Figure 2.34).

File	Edit	Data	Transform

  New ▶
  Open ▶
  Read ASCII Data...

  Close
  Save Data
  Save As...
  Export Chart...

  Display Data Info...
  Apply Data Dictionary...
  Apply Chart Template...

  Print...
  Printer Setup...
  Stop SPSS Processor   F3

  Exit

Figure 2.34 Selecting Read ASCII Data... from the File menu

This opens the Read ASCII Data File box (Figure 2.35), from which you choose the appropriate File Format, Directory and File Name. The fixed file format is one in which for all the cases every variable is in the same column locations, whereas in the freefield format only the order of the variables is consistent, with spaces acting as delimiters between variables. Only numeric and string data can be read in the freefield format.

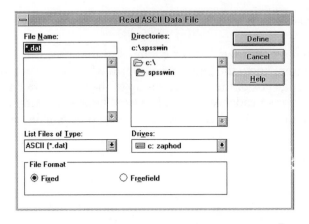

Figure 2.35 The Read ASCII Data File box

Then click the Define button to define the names, start and end columns, and data types for the variables.

3 CHOOSING A STATISTICAL TEST

This chapter provides a guide to choosing the right statistical test(s) to run in difference circumstances. However, this is not meant to be a replacement for a working knowledge of statistics and the reader is strongly urged to refer to a standard textbook of statistics for further information, including an understanding of why the tests chosen are the correct ones. The choice of appropriate statistical tests should be made before the research project is carried out and the data are collected; in other words, the research should be planned in advance.

Note that this chapter does not cover tests that are not considered in this book, such as multivariate tests.

Figure 3.1 is a flow diagram showing an overview of the choice of statistical test.

The first decision to make is whether you wish to look for a difference or a correlation between variables.

DIFFERENCES BETWEEN VARIABLES

Parametric data

In this case the data are measured on an interval or ratio scale (see Chapter 1) and fulfil the criteria for parametric tests (see Chapter 1).

If you wish to examine the difference between two such samples that are independent, the independent samples *t*-test can be used (see Chapter 6). If the two samples are related, the paired samples *t*-test should be used (see Chapter 6).

With more than two samples, an analysis of variance, or ANOVA, should be used (see Chapter 8), as follows.

A one-way ANOVA allows you to test the null hypothesis that the data are a sample from a population in which the mean of a test variable is equal in several independent groups of cases defined by a single grouping variable. The 'one-way' in the name of the ANOVA comes from the fact that the cases are allocated to the independent groups on the basis of values for that one test variable. There are no repeated measures.

Simple factorial ANOVA differs from one-way ANOVA in that it can handle several grouping variables (factors) simultaneously. With more than one factor, two types of 'treatment' effects (in ANOVA terminology) can occur:

1 *main effects*, which are the effects of the individual factors
2 an *interaction* between factors.

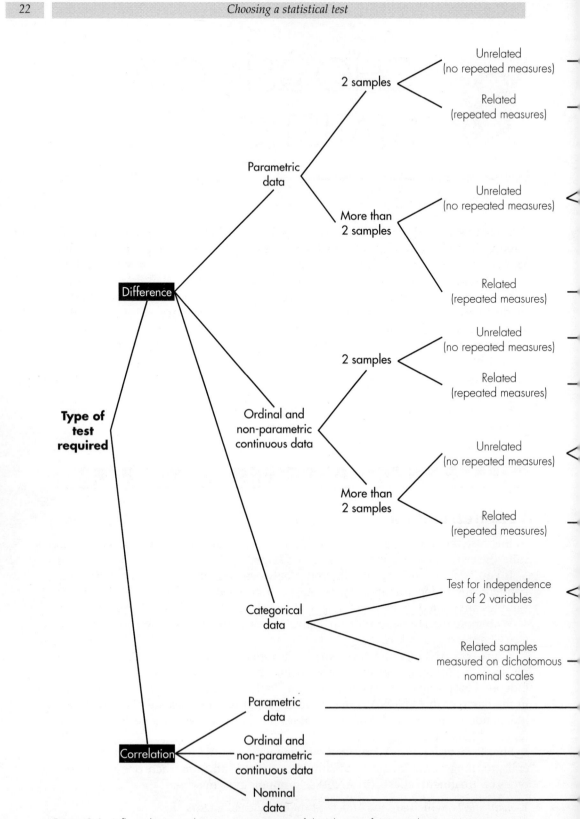

Figure 3.1 A flow diagram showing an overview of the choice of statistical test.

Independent samples
t-test
(Ch. 6)

Paired samples
t-test
(Ch. 6)

One grouping
variable
(factor)

One-way ANOVA
(Ch. 8)

More than
one grouping
variable (factor)

Control for
covariate(s)?

No —— Simple factorial ANOVA
(Ch. 8)

Yes —— General factorial ANOVA
(Ch. 8)

Repeated measures
ANOVA
(Ch. 8)

Mann–Whitney U test
(Ch. 6)

Wilcoxon matched-pairs test;
Sign test; or McNemar's test
(Ch 6)

One grouping variable
(factor)

Kruskal–Wallis test
(Ch 8)

More than one grouping
variable (factor)

Not available
in SPSS

Friedman test: or
Kendall's W test
(Ch.8)

One degree
of freedom

Fisher's exact probability test:
or chi-square test
(Ch.7)

More than one
degree of freedom

Chi-square test
(Ch.7)

Cochran's Q test
(Ch.8)

Pearson's product moment
correlation coefficient
(Ch.9)

Spearman's rank correlation;
or Kendall's tau-b
(Ch.9)

Phi coefficient; Cramer's V;
or the contingency coefficient
(Ch.9)

It is useful to run a general factorial ANOVA instead of a simple factorial ANOVA when you wish to control for covariates. (A covariate is a concomitant variable that is measured in addition to the dependent variable in ANOVA, and that represents an additional, uncontrolled for, source of variation in the dependent variable. For example, in a psychological study of visual perception, age may be a covariate if it has not been controlled for in the experiment.)

A repeated measures ANOVA is used to test hypotheses about the means of a dependent variable when the same dependent variable is measured on more than one occasion for each subject. Between-subjects variables are factors that subdivide the sample into discrete subgroups. Each subject can have only one value for a between-subjects factor. In contrast, within-subjects (repeated measures) variables are factors whose levels are all measured on the same subject. Mixed (split-plot) design experiments have a mixture of these two types of variables.

Ordinal and non-parametric continuous data

If you wish to examine the difference between two such samples that are independent, the Mann–Whitney U test can be used (see Chapter 6). If the two samples are related, SPSS offers the following three choices: the Wilcoxon matched-pairs test; the Sign test; and McNemar's test. Details of these choices are given in Chapter 6.

With more than two samples, a non-parametric ANOVA can be used (see Chapter 8), as follows.

The Kruskal–Wallis test is a non-parametric alternative to the one-way ANOVA and requires that the data be measured at least on an ordinal scale. The test statistic is calculated in the same way as the Mann–Whitney test statistic.

The median test is a non-parametric alternative to the one-way ANOVA that tests whether two or more samples are drawn from populations with the same median. It uses the chi-square statistic.

The Friedman test and Kendallís W test are non-parametric alternatives to the repeated measures ANOVA that are suitable for data measured on at least an ordinal scale.

Categorical data

For categorical data, that is, nominal (qualitative) data or ordinal data assigned to ordered categories, the chi-square test can be carried out to test for independence of two variables (see Chapter 7). For a given contingency table, the chi-square test should not be used if any cell has an expected frequency of less than one, or if more than 20 per cent of cells have expected frequencies of less than five. If these criteria are not met and the contingency table has just two rows and two columns, then Fisher's exact probability test can be carried out instead (Chapter 7). If the criteria are not met and there are more than two rows and/or columns, you can try to combine rows and columns so that the criteria are met.

Cochran's Q test is a non-parametric alternative to the repeated measures ANOVA that tests the null hypothesis that the proportion of cases in a particular category is the same for several dichotomous variables (Chapter 8). It is suitable for use when there are related samples measured on dichotomous (binary) nominal scales.

CORRELATION BETWEEN VARIABLES

Parametric data

In this case the data are measured on an interval or ratio scale (see Chapter 1) and fulfil the criteria for parametric tests (see Chapter 1).

If you wish to examine the correlation between two such samples, evaluate Pearson's product moment correlation coefficient (see Chapter 9). A linear regression equation can also be determined (see Chapter 10).

Ordinal and non-parametric continuous data

If you wish to examine the correlation between two such samples, either Spearman's rank correlation or Kendall's tau-b can be evaluated (see Chapter 9).

Nominal data

SPSS offers the following three measures of association based on the chi-square statistic: the phi coefficient; Cramér's V; and the contingency coefficient. These are described in Chapter 9.

4 EXPLORING DATA

A data distribution can be summarized by giving both a measure of its location, for example the mean, and a measure of its dispersion, for example the standard deviation. In addition, it is usually important to have an overview of the shape of the distribution when deciding which statistical tests can be applied.

NOMINAL AND ORDINAL DATA

Measures of central tendency

MODE

The mode of a distribution is the value of the observation occurring most frequently and can be used with all measurement scales.

	ageyr	level	downs	psych	epilepsy	causcpco	rx	unnatura	sex	va
1	86.335	sever	no	none	no	respiratory tract infection	no psych	0	mal	
2	82.335	mode	no	none	no	respiratory tract infection	no psych	0	mal	
3	65.970	sever	no	none	no	respiratory tract infection	no psych	0	mal	
4	82.151	sever	no	none	no	respiratory tract infection	no psych	0	mal	
5	86.324	mode	no	none	no	respiratory tract infection	no psych	0	mal	
6	72.541	mode	no	none	no	cerebrovascular	no psych	0	mal	
7	63.375	mode	yes	none	no	respiratory tract infection	no psych	0	mal	
8	19.349	mild	no	psych	no	suicide	no psych	hanging	mal	
9	72.686	mild	no	none	yes	cardiovascular disease	no psych	0	mal	
10	67.358	mild	no	mood	yes	cardiovascular disease	no psych	0	mal	
11	74.663	mode	no	none	no	other infection	no psych	0	mal	
12	60.248	mild	no	none	no	other infection	no psych	0	mal	
13	76.131	sever	no	none	no	respiratory tract infection	no psych	0	mal	

1:causcpco cp

SPSS Processor is ready

Figure 4.1   Highlighted nominal variable

The highlighted variable in Figure 4.1 is measured on a nominal scale and represents the cause of death for a certain sample of patients.

To determine the mode for this variable, this variable should be a recorded as a numeric variable with value labels corresponding to each of the categories. Open the Frequencies box as shown in Figure 4.2.

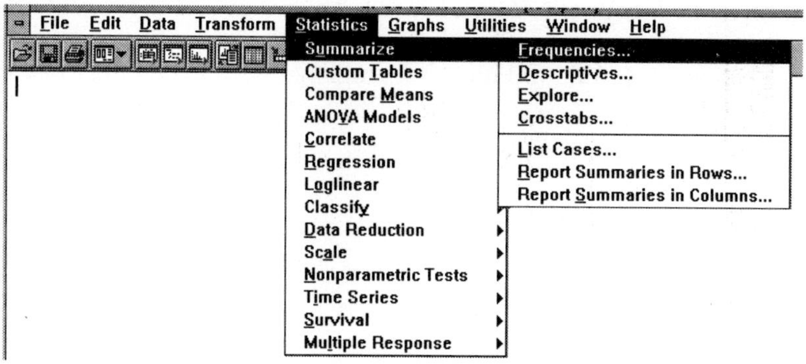

Figure 4.2 Opening the Frequencies box

In the Frequencies box, select the required variable (causcpco) and move it into the Variable(s) box by clicking the arrow button. If you do not require a frequency table, then deselect Display frequency tables (Figure 4.3).

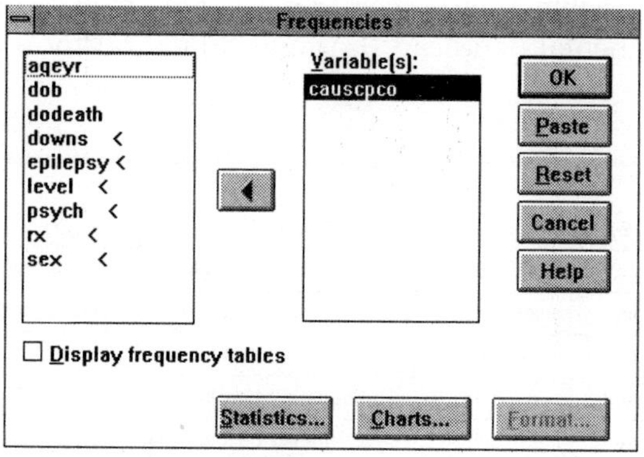

Figure 4.3 The Frequencies box

Click on the Statistics button to open the Frequencies: Statistics box. Select Mode under Central Tendency (Figure 4.4) and then click Continue.

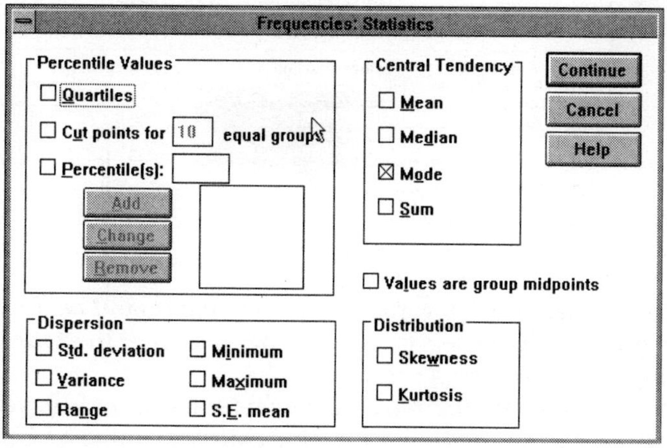

Figure 4.4 The Frequencies: Statistics box

On returning to the Frequencies box, click OK. This takes you to the Output screen where the value label corresponding to the mode is stated (in this case 8 = respiratory tract infection), as required (Figure 4.5), together with the number of valid and missing cases.

```
CAUSCPCO   cause of death


Mode              8.000


Valid cases       311       Missing cas
```

Figure 4.5 Output screen showing the value of the mode

MEDIAN

The median is the middle value of a set of observations ranked in order and can be used with measurement scales that are at least ordinal (that is, ordinal, interval or ratio).

The highlighted variable in Figure 4.6 is measured on an ordinal scale and represents the level of mental handicap (learning disability) for a certain sample of patients.

	ageyr	level	downs	psych	epilepsy	causcpco	rx	unnatura	sex
1	86.335	severe	no	none	no	respiratory tract infection	no psych	0	mal
2	82.335	moderate	no	none	no	respiratory tract infection	no psych	0	mal
3	65.970	severe	no	none	no	respiratory tract infection	no psych	0	mal
4	82.151	severe	no	none	no	respiratory tract infection	no psych	0	mal
5	86.324	moderate	no	none	no	respiratory tract infection	no psych	0	mal
6	72.541	moderate	no	none	no	cerebrovascular	no psych	0	mal
7	63.375	moderate	yes	none	no	respiratory tract infection	no psych	0	mal
8	19.349	mild	no	psych	no	suicide	no psych	hanging	mal
9	72.686	mild	no	none	yes	cardiovascular	no psych	0	mal
10	67.358	mild	no	mood	yes	cardiovascular	no psych	0	mal
11	74.663	moderate	no	none	no	other infection	no psych	0	mal
12	60.248	mild	no	none	no	other infection	no psych	0	mal
13	76.131	severe	no	none	no	respiratory tract infection	no psych	0	mal

1:level   3

SPSS Processor is ready

Figure 4.6 Highlighted ordinal variable

To determine the median for this variable, this variable should be a recorded as a numeric variable with value labels corresponding to each of the categories. Open the Frequencies box as shown above in Figure 4.2.

In the Frequencies box select the required variable (level) and move it into the Variable(s) box by clicking the arrow button. If you do not require a frequency table, then deselect Display frequency tables (Figure 4.7).

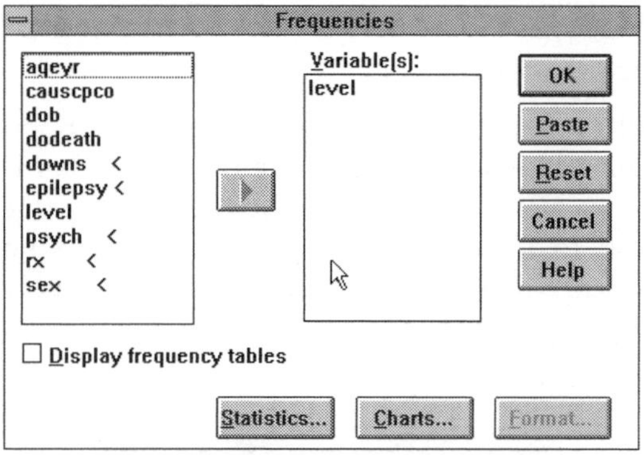

Figure 4.7 The Frequencies box

Click on the Statistics button to open the Frequencies: Statistics box. Select Median under Central Tendency (Figure 4.8) and then click Continue.

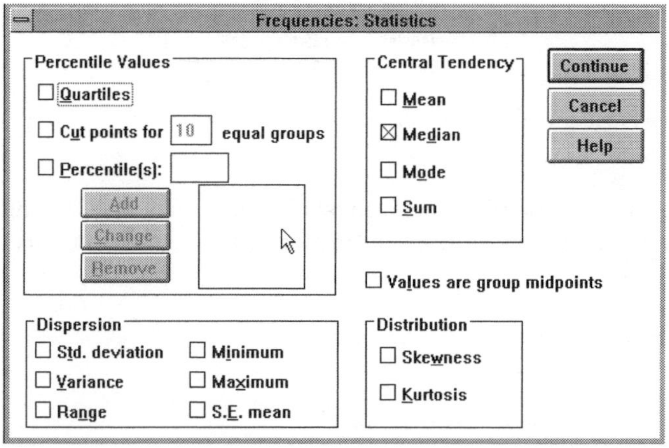

Figure 4.8 The Frequencies: Statistics box

On returning to the Frequencies box, click OK. This takes you to the Output screen where the value label corresponding to the median is stated (in this case 3 = severe mental retardation), as required (Figure 4.9), together with the number of valid and missing cases.

```
LEVEL       level of handicap


Median        3.000


Valid cases      325      Missing cases      0
```

Figure 4.9 Output screen showing the value of the median

Distribution shape

DIAGRAMMATIC REPRESENTATION

Nominal and ordinal data can be represented by bar charts. Suppose we wish to represent the nominal variable highlighted in Figure 4.1 as a bar chart. First open the Frequencies box (Figure 4.2) and select the required variable (Figure 4.3). Then click on the Charts... button, to open the Frequencies: Charts box. Choose the Bar chart(s) radio button and decide whether you would like the axis label display to be in frequencies or percentages (Figure 4.10).

```
┌─────────────────────────────────────────────┐
│ ▬│          Frequencies: Charts              │
├─────────────────────────────────────────────┤
│  ┌─Chart Type──────────┐   ┌──────────┐      │
│  │  ○ None             │   │ Continue │      │
│  │  ⦿ Bar chart(s)     │   └──────────┘      │
│  │  ○ Histogram(s)     │   ┌──────────┐      │
│  │                     │   │  Cancel  │      │
│  │  ☐ With norm curve  │   └──────────┘      │
│  └─────────────────────┘   ┌──────────┐      │
│                            │   Help   │      │
│  ┌─Axis Label Display──────└──────────┘──┐   │
│  │  ⦿ Frequencies    ○ Percentages      │   │
│  └──────────────────────────────────────┘   │
└─────────────────────────────────────────────┘
```

Figure 4.10 The Frequencies: Charts box

Click on Continue and then, in the Frequencies box, click on OK. This takes you to the Output window, where you are informed that the bar chart has been created (Figure 4.11).

```
CAUSCPCO   cause of death


Hi-Res Chart  # 1:Bar chart of cause of death

Valid cases      311      Missing cases      14



◄│
```

○ Chart Carousel

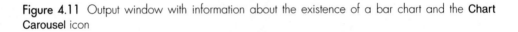

SPSS Processor is ready

Figure 4.11 Output window with information about the existence of a bar chart and the **Chart Carousel** icon

Also present is the Chart Carousel icon (see Figure 4.11) which should now be double clicked (with the left mouse button) to take you to the **Chart Carousel** containing the required bar chart (Figure 4.12).

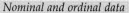

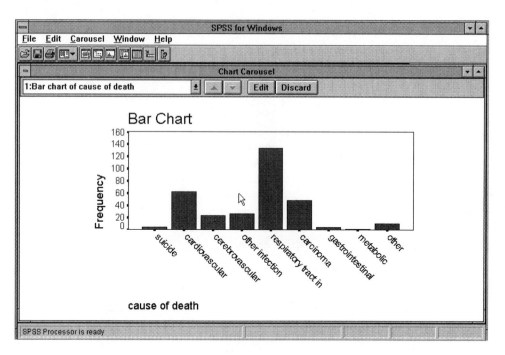

Figure 4.12 Bar chart

Objects in the Chart Carousel can be edited by clicking on the Edit button and then using the mouse and toolbar.

An alternative way of obtaining a bar chart is from the Graphs menu (Figure 4.13).

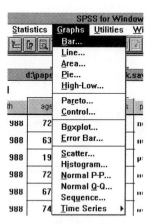

Figure 4.13 Selecting bar charts from the Graphs menu

This opens the Bar Charts box (Figure 4.14).

Select the type of chart you want and then click Define to take you to the Define Simple Bar box, in which you make the appropriate choices (see Figure 4.15) and then click OK to obtain the bar chart as before.

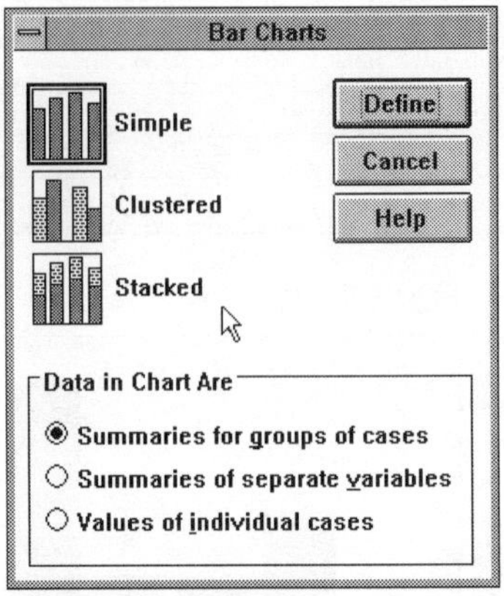

Figure 4.14 The Bar Charts box

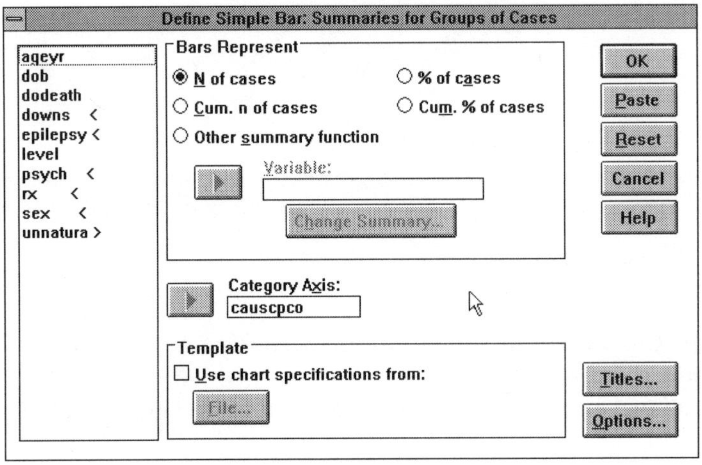

Figure 4.15 The Define Simple Bar box

Nominal and ordinal data can also be represented by pie charts (pie diagrams). Suppose that we wish to represent the ordinal variable highlighted in Figure 4.6 as a pie chart. From the Graphs menu select Pie (Figure 4.16).

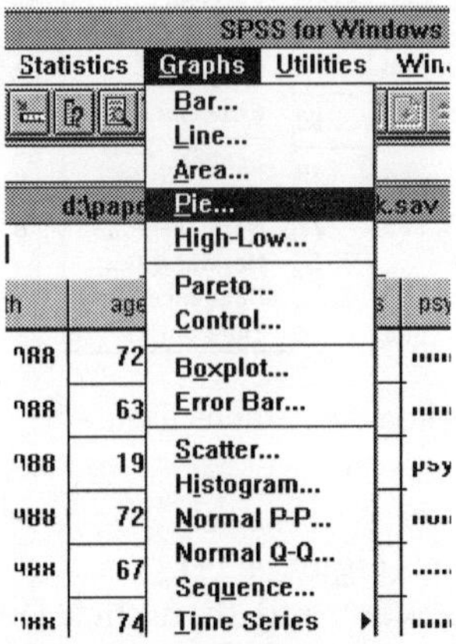

Figure 4.16 Selecting pie charts from the Graphs menu

This leads to the Pie Charts box, in which, after selecting the appropriate radio button (Figure 4.17), you should click on Define.

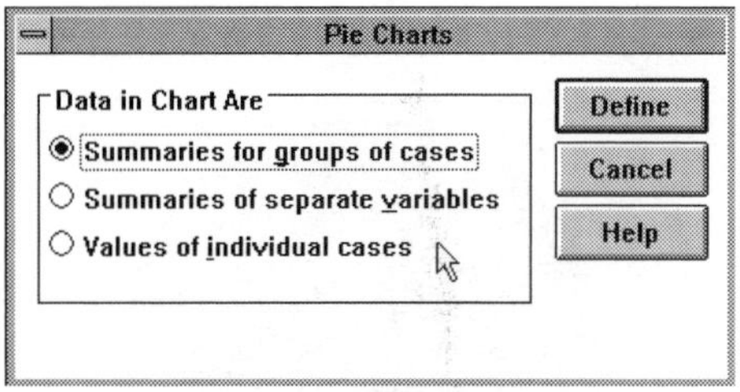

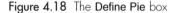

Figure 4.17 The Pie Charts box

This opens the Define Pie box in which you make the appropriate choices (see Figure 4.18); in this case we have opted for the slices to represent percentages.

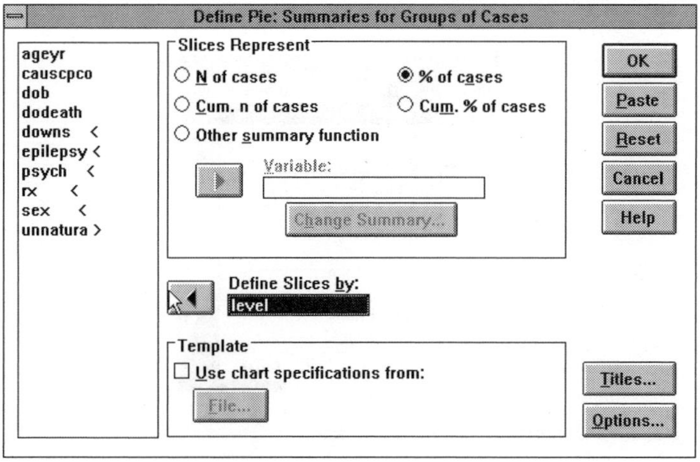

Figure 4.18 The Define Pie box

Clicking OK then takes you to the Chart Carousel and the required pie chart (Figure 4.19).

(The default SPSS settings will probably generate a pie chart using difference colours for the difference slices, but the colours have been edited in Figure 4.19 for the purposes of monochrome reproduction in this book.) As usual, diagrams in the Chart Carousel can be edited by clicking the Edit button (not shown in Figure 4.19 which is already in edit format). For example, to display the actual percentages, first select Options from the Chart menu, as shown in Figure 4.20.

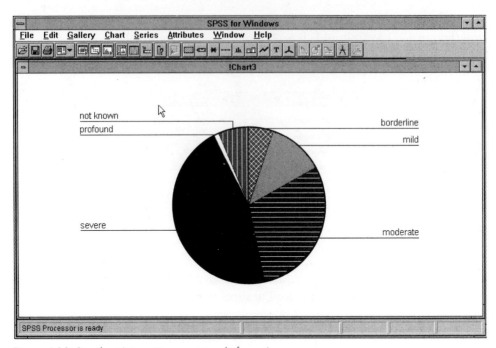

Figure 4.19 Pie chart (**Chart Carousel** in edit format)

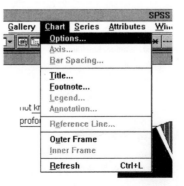

Figure 4.20 Selecting **Options** from the **Chart** menu

This opens the **Pie Options** box, in which in this case you wish to select **Percents** (in addition to **Text**), as shown in Figure 4.21.

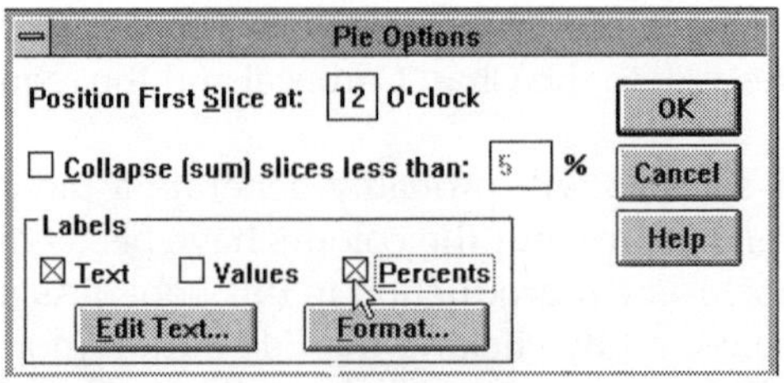

Figure 4.21 The **Pie Options** box

Clicking on OK returns you to the Chart Carousel, and the revised version of the pie chart shown in Figure 4.22.

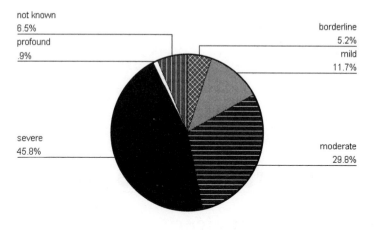

Figure 4.22 Pie chart with percentages

FREQUENCIES

Tables of frequencies can be obtained by opening the Frequencies box as shown in Figure 4.2 above. Click on Display frequency tables. For example, to obtain a frequency table for the ordinal variable highlighted in Figure 4.6, the Frequencies box would appear as shown in Figure 4.23.

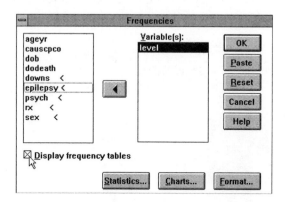

Figure 4.23 Obtaining a frequency table

Clicking on OK takes you to the Output window where the required frequency table appears (Figure 4.24).

```
LEVEL      level of handicap


                                                Valid      Cum
Value Label                 Value  Frequency  Percent  Percent  Percent

borderline                    0        17       5.2      5.2      5.2
mild                          1        38      11.7     11.7     16.9
moderate                      2        97      29.8     29.8     46.8
severe                        3       149      45.8     45.8     92.6
profound                      4         3       .9       .9      93.5
not known                     9        21       6.5      6.5     100.0
                                     -------   -------  -------
                            Total     325     100.0    100.0


Valid cases      325     Missing cases      0
```

Figure 4.24 A frequency table

INTERVAL AND RATIO DATA

Measures of central tendency

MODE AND MEDIAN

See above.

ARITHMETIC MEAN

The (arithmetic) mean is the average value of a distribution and can be used for continuous data, that is, data measured on an interval or ratio scale.

The highlighted variable (ageyr) in Figure 4.25 is measured on a ratio scale and represents the age at death for a certain sample of patients.

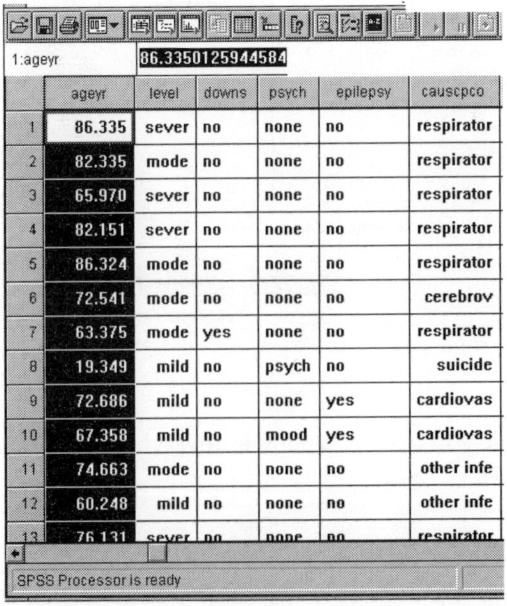

	ageyr	level	downs	psych	epilepsy	causcpco
1:ageyr	86.3350125944584					
1	86.335	sever	no	none	no	respirator
2	82.335	mode	no	none	no	respirator
3	65.970	sever	no	none	no	respirator
4	82.151	sever	no	none	no	respirator
5	86.324	mode	no	none	no	respirator
6	72.541	mode	no	none	no	cerebrov
7	63.375	mode	yes	none	no	respirator
8	19.349	mild	no	psych	no	suicide
9	72.686	mild	no	none	yes	cardiovas
10	67.358	mild	no	mood	yes	cardiovas
11	74.663	mode	no	none	no	other infe
12	60.248	mild	no	none	no	other infe
13	76.131	sever	no	none	no	respirator

SPSS Processor is ready

Figure 4.25 Highlighted continuous (ratio) variable

To determine the mean for this variable, select Descriptives from the Statistics menu, as shown in Figure 4.26.

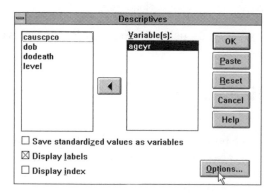

Transform	Statistics	Graphs	Utilities	Window	Help
	Summarize		Frequencies...		
	Custom Tables		Descriptives...		
5012594456	Compare Means		Explore...		
downs	ANOVA Models		Crosstabs...		
	Correlate		List Cases...		
r no n	Regression		Report Summaries in Rows...		
: no n	Loglinear		Report Summaries in Columns...		
	Classify				
r no n	Data Reduction ▶		no psych	0	mal
r no n	Scale ▶		no psych	0	mal
	Nonparametric Tests ▶				
: no n	Time Series ▶		no psych	0	mal
	Survival ▶				
: no n	Multiple Response ▶		no psych	0	mal

Figure 4.26 Selecting Descriptives

This opens the Descriptives box shown in Figure 4.27, in which the required variable (ageyr) has been selected.

Figure 4.27 The Descriptives box

Click on Options to open the Descriptives: Options box, in which Mean should be selected (Figure 4.28).

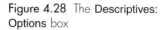

Figure 4.28 The Descriptives: Options box

Clicking on Continue returns you to the Descriptives box. Clicking on OK takes you to the Output window where the required mean (68.38 years) appears (Figure 4.29).

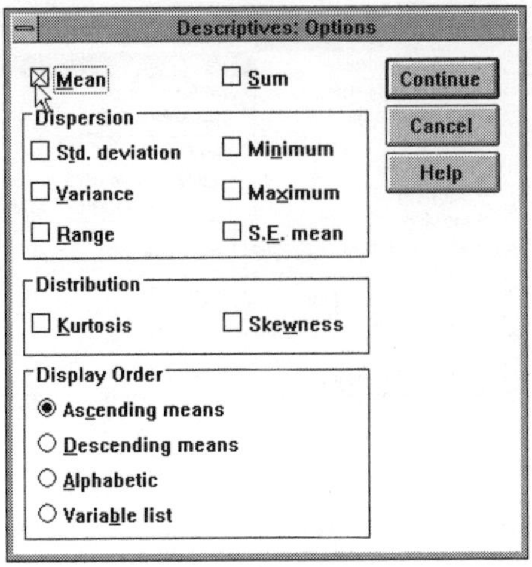

Figure 4.29 Output screen showing the value of the mean

The mean can also be obtained by using the Frequencies: Statistics box (Figure 4.8 or Figure 4.31).

Measures of dispersion

RANGE

The range is the difference between the smallest and largest values in a distribution and can be used for data measured on an interval or ratio scale.

The range can be obtained by selecting Range in the Descriptives: Options box shown in Figure 4.28. The resulting Output is shown in Figure 4.30 (range = 84.96 years).

```
Number of valid observations (listwise) =        307.00

                         Valid
Variable      Range        N   Label

AGEYR        84.96       307   age in years
```

Figure 4.30 Output screen showing the value of the range

To obtain the values of the minimum and maximum, these should be selected in the Descriptives: Options box.

MEASURES RELATING TO QUANTILES

The interquartile range is the difference between the third and the first quartile.

To obtain the interquartile range for the variable ageyr (Figure 4.25) open the Frequencies box as shown in Figure 4.2. Click on Statistics to obtain the Frequencies: Statistics box, in which Quartiles should be selected (Figure 4.31).

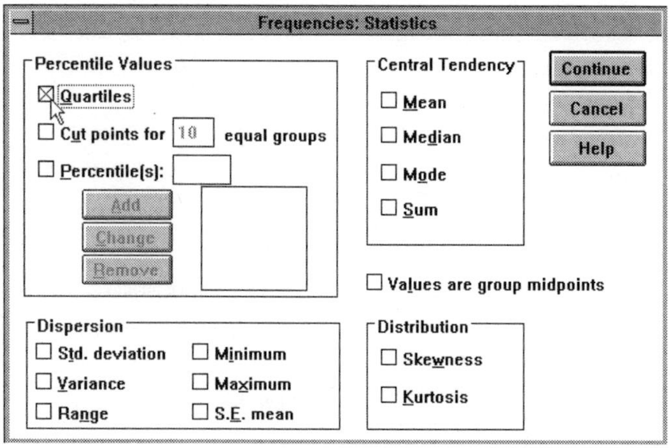

Figure 4.31 The **Frequencies: Statistics** box – obtaining quartiles

Click on **Continue** to return to the **Frequencies** box and then on **OK**. The resulting Output is shown in Figure 4.32, in which the values of the first quartile (25.00 percentile), median or second quartile (50.00 percentile) and third quartile (75.00 percentile) are given as 60.095, 72.821 and 81.968 years, respectively. The interquartile range is obtained by subtracting the value of the first quartile from that of the third quartile, and in this case is 81.968 − 60.095 = 21.873 years.

```
AGEYR     age in years


Percentile    Value      Percentile    Value      Percentile    Value

  25.00      60.095        50.00      72.821        75.00      81.968

Valid cases      307     Missing cases      18
```

Figure 4.32 **Output** screen showing the values of the quartiles

The semi-interquartile range or quartile deviation is one-half of the difference between the third and the first quartile. It is calculated by subtracting the value of the first quartile from that of the third quartile, as above, and then dividing the result by two. With the variable ageyr (Figure 4.25) the semi-interquartile range or quartile deviation = 21.873/2 = 10.9365 years.

The 10 to 90 percentile range, or interdecile range, is the difference between the 90th and 10th (per)centiles, or equivalently, between the ninth and first deciles.

To obtain the 10 to 90 percentile (interdecile) range for the variable ageyr (Figure 4.25) open the **Frequencies** box as shown in Figure 4.2 on page 00. Click on **Statistics** to obtain the **Frequencies: Statistics** box, in which **Percentiles** should be selected. Add in 10 and 90 (Figure 4.33).

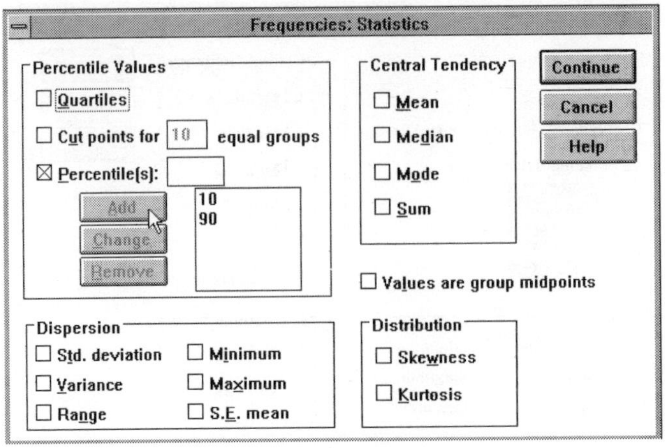

Figure 4.33 The **Frequencies: Statistics** box – obtaining the 10 to 90 percentile (interdecile) range

Click on **Continue** to return to the **Frequencies** box and then on **OK**. The resulting
Output is shown in Figure 4.34, in which the values of the 10th and 90th percentiles
are respectively given as 38.994 and 87.496 years. The 10 to 90 percentile (interdecile)
range is obtained by subtracting the value of the 10th percentile from the 90th percentile, and in this case is equal to 87.496 – 38.994 = 48.502 years.

```
AGEYR      age in years


Percentile     Value     Percentile     Value

   10.00      38.994       90.00       87.496

Valid cases     307     Missing cases     18
```

Figure 4.34 **Output** screen showing the values of the 10th and 90th percentiles

STANDARD DEVIATION

The standard deviation of a distribution is a measure of dispersion based on deviations from the mean (which are squared, summed, and (approximately) averaged
and then the square root is taken), has the same units as the original observations,
and can be used for data measured on an interval or ratio scale.

To obtain the standard deviation for the variable ageyr (Figure 4.25) open the
Descriptives: Options box as shown in Figures 4.26 to 4.28 above. Select **Std. deviation**
(Figure 4.35).

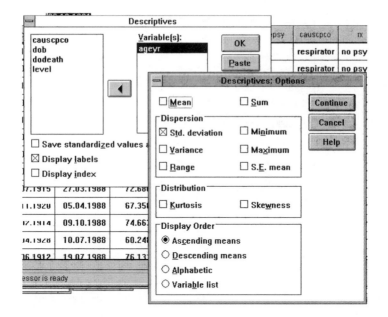

Figure 4.35 The **Descriptives: Options** box – obtaining the standard deviation

Click on **Continue** to return to the **Descriptives** box and then on **OK**. The resulting Output is shown in Figure 4.36, in which the value of the standard deviation is given as 18.24 years.

```
Number of valid observations (listwise) =      307.00

                          Valid
Variable    Std Dev        N   Label

AGEYR        18.24        307   age in years
```

Figure 4.36 Output screen showing the value of the standard deviation

VARIANCE

The variance is the square of the standard deviation, has units that are the square of those of the original observations, and can be used for data measured on an interval or ratio scale.

To obtain the variance for the variable ageyr (Figure 4.25) open the **Descriptives: Options** box as shown in Figures 4.26 to 4.28 above. Select **Variance** (Figure 4.37).

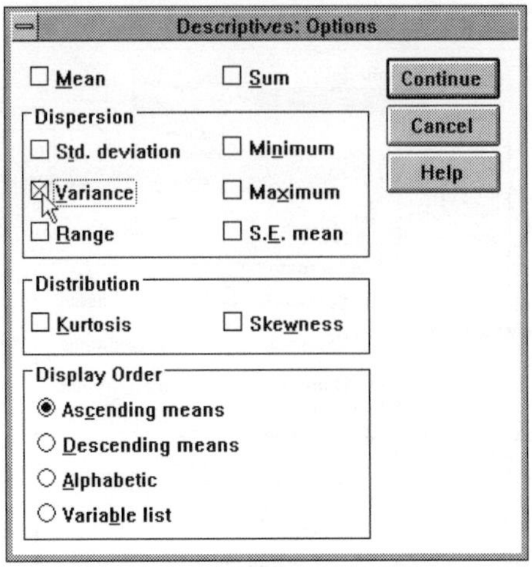

Figure 4.37 The **Descriptives: Options** box – obtaining the variance

Click on **Continue** to return to the **Descriptives** box and then on **OK**. The resulting Output is shown in Figure 4.38, in which the value of the variance is given as 332.83 year^2.

```
Number of valid observations (listwise) =        307.00

                             Valid
Variable    Variance        N   Label

AGEYR        332.83       307  age in years
```

Figure 4.38 **Output** screen showing the value of the variance

Distribution shape

DIAGRAMMATIC REPRESENTATION

Interval and ordinal data can be represented by histograms. Suppose that we wish to represent the ratio variable highlighted in Figure 4.25 as a histogram. First select Histogram from the Graphics menu (Figure 4.39).

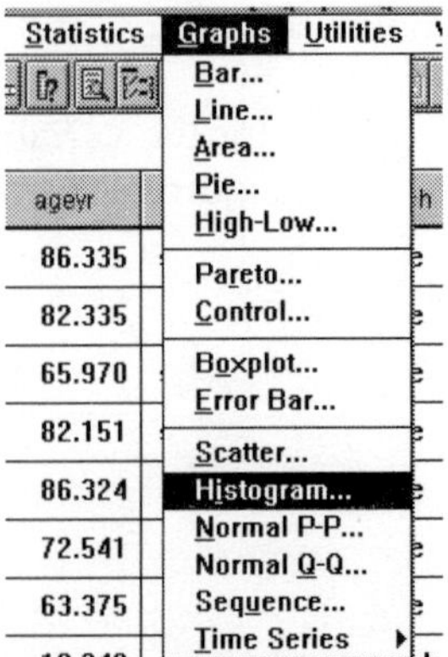

Figure 4.39 Selecting histogram from the **Graphs** menu

In the Histogram box select the required variable (Figure 4.40).

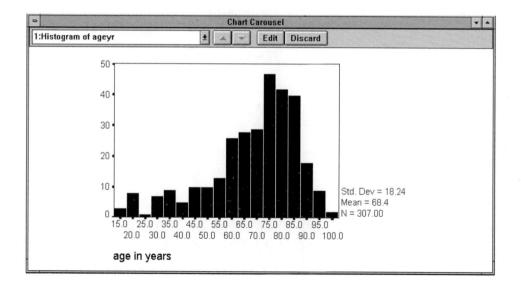

Figure 4.40 The Histogram box

Click on OK. The histogram is in the Chart Carousel (Figure 4.41) and can be edited using the Edit functions.

Figure 4.41 Histogram

A stem-and-leaf diagram, which can also be used to represent continuous (interval or ratio) data, differs from a histogram in that it allows all the individual data to be shown. To represent the continuous (ratio) variable highlighted in Figure 4.25 as a stem-and-leaf diagram, first select Explore from the Statistics menu (Figure 4.42).

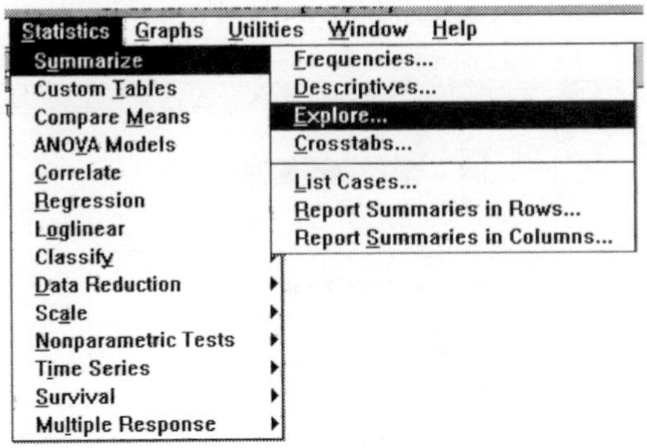

Figure 4.42 Selecting Explore

In the resulting Explore box, select the required variable and the Display Plots radio button, as shown in Figure 4.43.

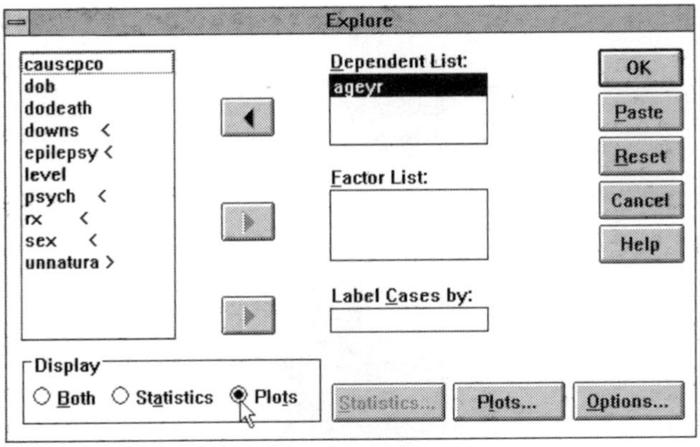

Figure 4.43 The Explore box

Clicking on Plots... opens the Explore: Plots box, in which Stem-and-leaf should be selected (Figure 4.44).

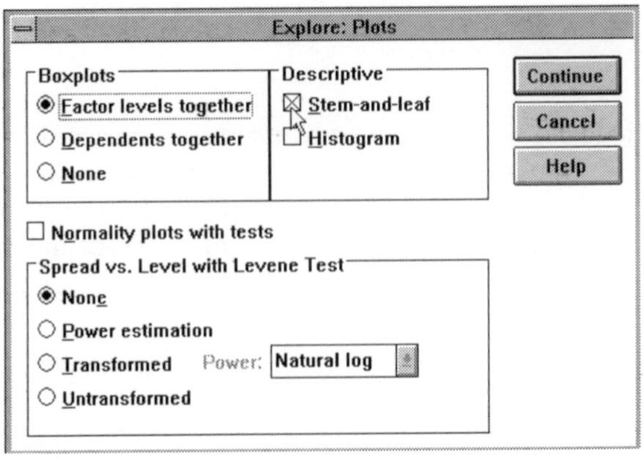

Figure 4.44 The Explore: Plots box

Click on Continue and then, on returning to the Explore box, click OK. The required
stem-and-leaf diagram appears in the Output window (Figure 4.45).

```
        AGEYR       age in years

    Valid cases:       307.0   Missing cases:      18.0   Percent missing:    5.5


    Frequency    Stem & Leaf

        12.00 Extremes      (16), (16), (17), (19), (19), (21), (25)
         4.00      2 .  99
         9.00      3 *  0344&
         7.00      3 .  689
         7.00      4 *  344&
         9.00      4 .  789&
         9.00      5 *  003&
        18.00      5 .  55668999&
        31.00      6 *  00001111223344
        27.00      6 .  555677888999
        43.00      7 *  00011222222333333444
        37.00      7 .  556666777777788999
        48.00      8 *  000111111122222233333444
        27.00      8 .  555666777999&
        15.00      9 *  0111234
         2.00      9 .  6
         2.00     10 *  0

    Stem width:    10.000
    Each leaf:      2 case(s)


    & denotes fractional leaves.
```

Figure 4.45 Stem-and-leaf diagram

The above procedure also produces a box plot (box-and-whisker plot) in the Chart
Carousel (Figure 4.46). In this plot the upper and lower boundaries of the box are
the upper and lower quartiles, respectively. The box length is the interquartile range.
The thick line inside the box is the median. The vertical lines from the box (whiskers)
extend to the smallest and largest observations (marked with X) that are less than
one interquartile range from the end of the box. O (outlier) marks points outside this
range but less than 1.5 interquartile distances away. E marks points more than 1.5
interquartile ranges from the end of the box.

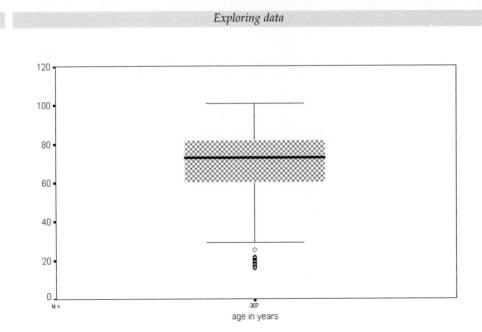

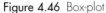

Figure 4.46 Box-plot

FREQUENCIES

Obtaining frequency tables has been described above (Figures 4.23 and 4.24.

TESTS OF NORMALITY

As mentioned in Chapter 3, it is often important to test whether the sample data come from a normal distribution. Suppose that we wish to carry out such a test for the variable (ageyr) highlighted in Figure 4.25. In the Explore box (see Figure 4.42 for details of how to select it) select the required variable, select the Display Both radio button, and click Plots... (Figure 4.47).

Figure 4.47 The Explore box with the Plots... button about to be clicked

In the resulting Explore: Plots box, select Normality plots with tests to display normal probability and detrended normal probability plots (and deselect Boxplots), as shown in Figure 4.48. This option also calculates the Kolmogorov–Smirnov statistic, with a Lilliefors significance level for testing normality; the Shapiro–Wilks statistic is also calculated if the sample size is small.

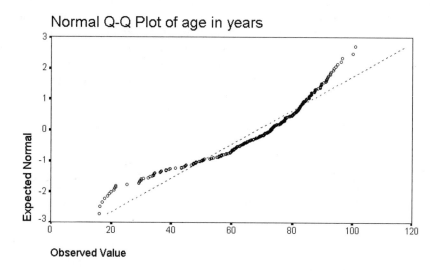

Figure 4.48 The Explore: Plots box – selecting Normality plots with tests

Click on Continue and then, in the Explore box, on OK. In the Chart Carousel two plots are produced. The Normal Q–Q (Quantile–Quantile) plot shows the oberved values of the variable (along the horizontal axis) plotted against the corresponding values predicted if the data are from a standard normal distribution (along the vertical axis). If the data are indeed from a normal distribution, then the points in this plot would be expected to cluster around the dotted straight line shown in Figure 4.49.

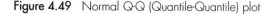

Figure 4.49 Normal Q-Q (Quantile-Quantile) plot

In this case there appears to be a definite deviation from the straight line. The other plot produced is a detrended normal plot. This is a plot of the differences between the observed values and the corresponding predicted values if the sample is from a normal distribution. If the sample is indeed from a normal distribution, then the points should cluster in a horizontal band around zero and there should not be a pattern; this is not the case for the detrended normal Q–Q plot shown in Figure 4.50.

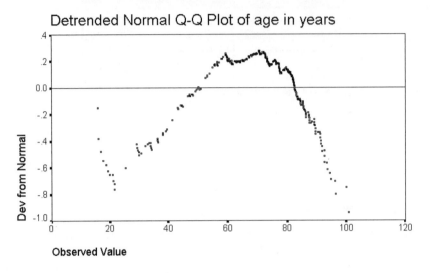

Figure 4.50 Detrended normal Q-Q plot

In the Output window, the value of the Kolmogorov–Smirnov statistic, with the Lilliefors correction applied, is given. This is a test of normality based on the absolute value of the maximum difference between the observed cumulative distribution and that expected based on the assumption of normality (Figure 4.51). If the significance level (highlighted in Figure 4.51) is too small, as in this case, then the normality assumption is an unreasonable one (and vice versa). That is, in this case, the data should not be taken as having a normal distribution. In such a case, if you wish to use a statistical test requiring the assumption of normality (see the previous chapter), then you may wish to consider using data transformation, described in the next chapter.

	Statistic	df	Significance
K-S (Lilliefors)	.1095	307	.0000

Figure 4.51 Output screen showing the value of the Kolmogorov–Smirnov statistic, with the Lilliefors correction applied; the significance level is highlighted

5 DATA TRANSFORMATION AND SELECTION

DATA TRANSFORMATION

Data transformation involves changing the values of a variable. This may be carried out for a number of reasons, such as correcting coding errors, modify the coding scheme, creating new variables, constructing an index, or, as seen at the end of the last chapter, to alter the distribution of a variable so that it better matches another one, such as the normal distribution. An important feature of SPSS is that there is a choice between transforming an existing variable; or keeping the existing variable and creating a new variable (the transformed one); or choosing not to save the transformation at all (either by opening a new data file or exiting SPSS without saving the transformed variable).

Types of data transformation

In SPSS for Windows the following types of data transformation are available:

- Recode – discrete values are assigned to a variable based on its current values
- Compute – data values are computed according to the formula entered
- Automatic recode – the consecutive positive integers 1, 2, 3, 4, ... are automatically assigned to a new variable
- Count – a new variable is created that states for each case how many times specified values occur in other variables
- Random number seed – this sets the seed used by the pseudo-random number generator to a specific value, so that you can reproduce a sequence of pseudo-random number. (the random-number seed changes each time SPSS generates a random number for use in transformations)
- Rank cases – rank scores are created
- Create time series – new time series are created.

Descriptions of how to use certain of these transformations follow.

Recoding

In Figure 4.25 in the previous chapter, the continuous variable ageyr represents the age of death of a certain sample of patients. Suppose we wish to recode these ages into a separate categorical variable in which the categories are each three decades (0 up to but not including 30 years; 30 up to 60 years; and so on). Select Recode Into Different Variables..., as shown in Figure 5.1.

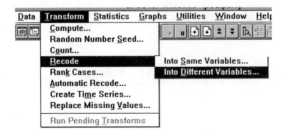

Figure 5.1 Selecting Recode

In the resulting Recode into Different Variables box, select the required variable (ageyr), type a name for the new categorical variable (ageyrcat) into the Output Variable Name box, and then click Change, as shown in Figure 5.2.

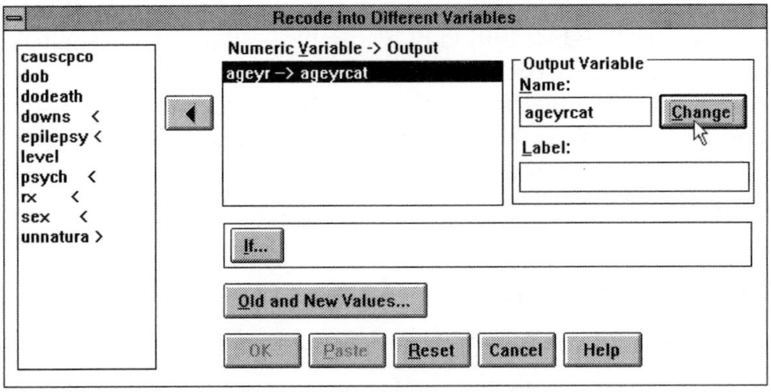

Figure 5.2 The Recode into Different Variables box

Next, click Old and New Values... to open the Recode into Different Variables: Old and New Values box. For the first category, select the Range radio button in the Old Value group and then enter 0 through 29.999 (for 0 up to 30 years). This will correspond to the category 1, which should therefore be entered in the New Value group, as shown in Figure 5.3.

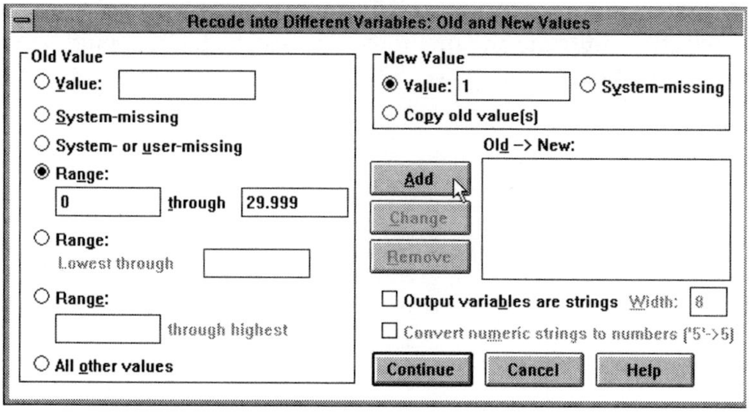

Figure 5.3 The Recode into Different Variables: Old and New Values box

Clicking Add then results in Figure 5.4.

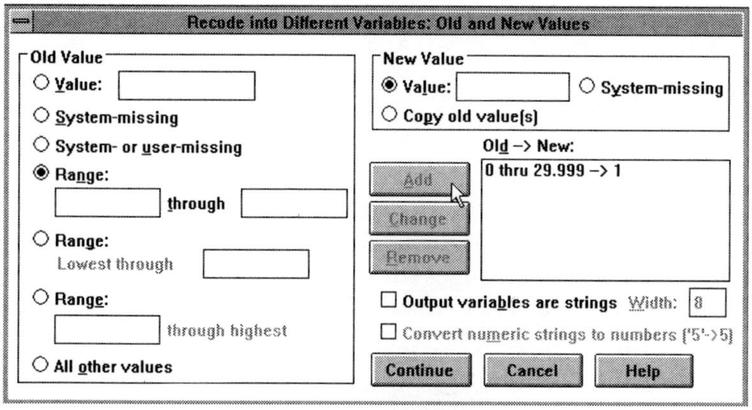

Figure 5.4 Partially completed Recode into Different Variables: Old and New Values box

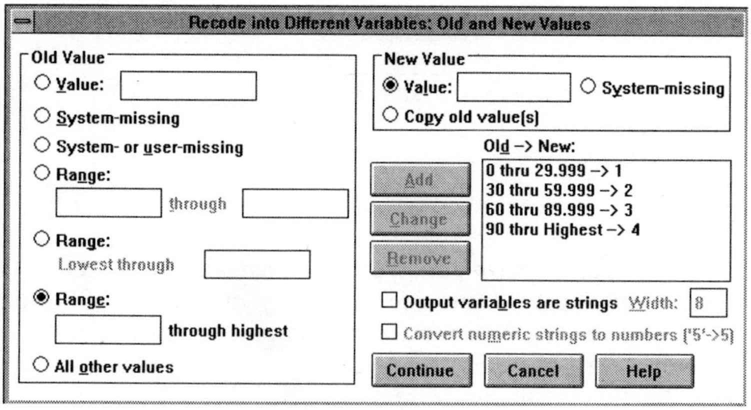

Figure 5.5 Completed Recode into Different Variables: Old and New Values box

The completed box is shown in Figure 5.5.

Click **Continue** to return to the previous box, in which **OK** should be clicked for the data transformation to take place. This can be checked in the data file (Figure 5.6).

ageyr	ageyrcat
86.335	3
82.335	3
65.970	3
82.151	3
86.324	3
72.541	3
63.375	3
19.349	1
72.686	3
67.358	3
74.663	3
60.248	3

Figure 5.6 Data file with recoded variable (ageyrcat) and original variable (ageyr)

Computing variables

Suppose we wished to convert the ages (in years) in the previous example (ageyr highlighted in Figure 4.25) into ages expressed as months. We will save the transformed data as a new variable, agemonth. Select **Compute...**, as shown in Figure 5.7.

Data	**Transform**	**Statistics**	**Graph**o
	Compute...		
	Random Number Seed...		
	Count...		
	Recode	▶	
	Rank Cases...		
	Automatic Recode...		
	Create Time Series...		
	Replace Missing Values...		
	Run Pending Transforms		

Figure 5.7 Selecting **Compute...**

In the resulting **Compute Variable** box, type in the name of the target variable (agemonth), click the **Type&Label** button to make any required modifications to the target variable, and use the **Numeric Expression** part of the box to construct the required formula (using the arrow buttons to paste variables and functions as required). The functions available are shown in the Appendix.

The calculator pad operators available are shown in Table 5.1.

Table 5.1 Calculator pad operators

Operator	Function
+	Add
-	Subtract
*	Multiply
/	Divide
**	Raise to power
<	Less than
<=	Less than or equal to
=	Equal to
&	And
~	Not
>	Greater than
>=	Greater than or equal to
~=	Not equal to
|	Or
()	Grouping parentheses

In our example, the formula required is agemonth = ageyr*12, as shown in Figure

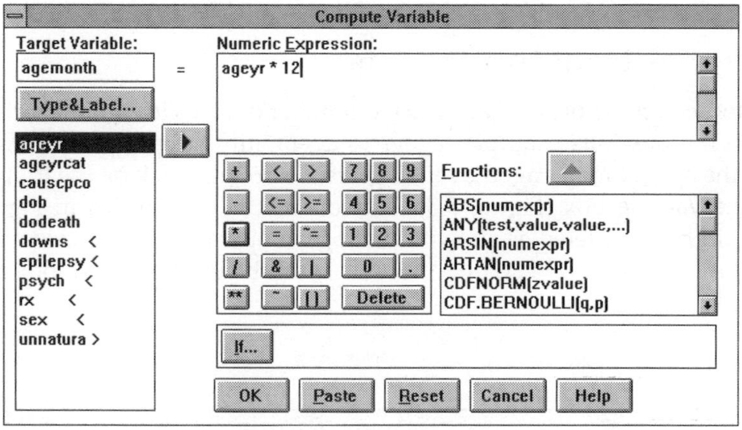

Figure 5.8 The Compute Variable box

Click on **OK** for the data transformation to take place. This can be checked in the data file (Figure 5.9).

ageyr	agemonth
86.335	1036.02
82.335	988.02
65.970	791.64
82.151	985.82
86.324	1035.89
72.541	870.50
63.375	760.50
19.349	232.19
72.686	872.24
67.358	808.30
74.663	895.96
60.248	722.98

Figure 5.9 Data file with computed variable (agemonth) and original variable (ageyr)

The compute function is particularly useful for carrying out transformations such as taking the logarithm (LG10 or LN) or square root (SQRT) when trying to make the distribution of a variable more closely match the normal distribution.

Conditional transformations

You can choose to transform only a selected number of cases in a given variable. For instance, in the previous example (ageyr to agemonth) suppose we wish only to transform the ages of males aged over 50 years. To do this, click on the If... button in the Compute Variable box (Figure 5.8). This opens the box shown in Figure 5.10, which should be completed as shown. The logical operators of the calculator pad, shown in Table 5.1 (<, <=, =, &, ~, >, >=, ~=, |) can be used to build logical operations.

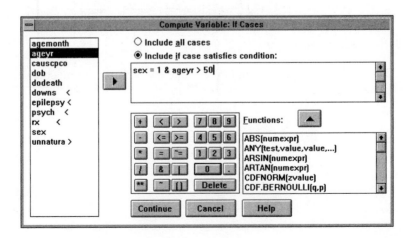

Figure 5.10 Compute Variable: If Cases box

Clicking on Continue returns you to the Compute Variable box, in which clicking OK allows the conditional transformation to take place.

DATA SELECTION

In order to use only selected cases, choose Select Cases, as shown in Figure 5.11.

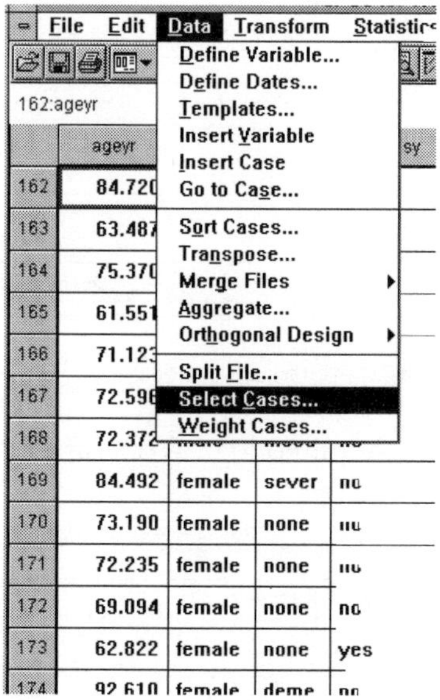

Figure 5.11 Selecting Select Cases

This opens the Select Cases box. Suppose we wanted to select males who had died at or over the age of 70 years in the previous example (ageyr; Figure 4.25). In the Select Cases box choose the If condition is satisfied radio button. If you wish the selection to be temporary, also choose the Filtered radio button; whereas if you wish the selection to be permanent, choose Deleted. Then click on the If... button shown in Figure 5.12.

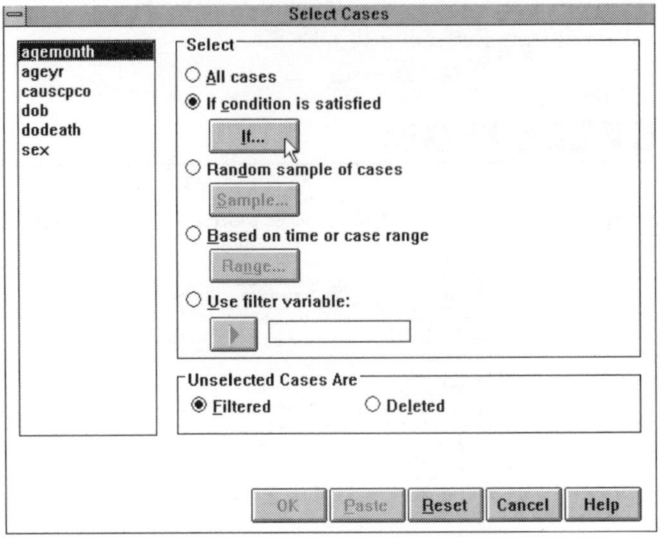

Figure 5.12 The Select Cases box

In the next box, construct the required logical operation (Figure 5.13).

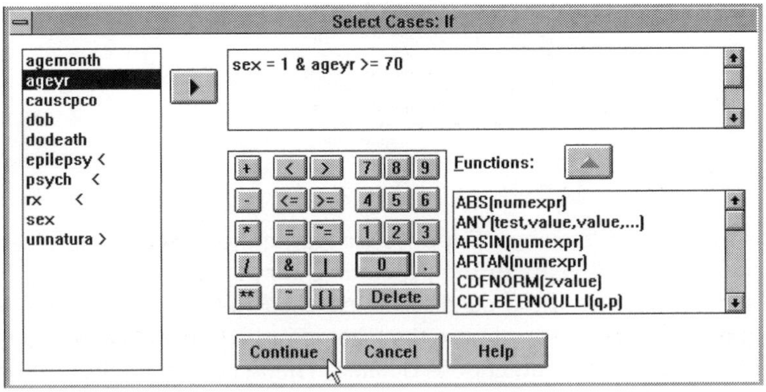

Figure 5.13 The Select Cases: If box

Click on Continue, and then on OK in the Select Cases box. The data file window confirms that the required selection has been made, with the case numbers of deselected cases being crossed, as shown in Figure 5.14.

	ageyr	sex
162	84.720	male
163	63.487	male
164	75.370	male
165	61.551	male
166	71.123	male
167	72.596	male
168	72.372	male
169	84.492	female
170	73.190	female
171	72.235	female
172	69.094	female
173	62.822	female

Figure 5.14 Data file with selected cases

6 COMPARING TWO SAMPLE AVERAGES

PARAMETRIC TESTS

The t-test is used for testing the null hypothesis that two population means are equal when the variable being investigated has a normal distribution in each population and the population variances are equal. SPSS automatically checks that the variances of the two groups are not significantly different, and if they are, the program gives adjusted probabilities corresponding to the value of t. Before carrying out a t-test, therefore, you should check that the data come from normal distributions (see Chapter 4); it is a useful step to plot the data.

Independent samples t-test

This procedure tests the null hypothesis that the data are a sample from a population in which the mean of a test variable is equal in two independent (unrelated) groups of cases.

Suppose we wish to test the null hypothesis, at the 5% level of significance, that there is no difference between the population mean ages of the males and females in the data file shown in Figure 6.1.

	age	sex
1	22.9	male
2	23.3	male
3	20.6	male
4	22.3	male
5	22.6	male
6	25.1	male
7	47.8	male
8	32.8	female
9	37.4	male
10	20.8	male
11	43.0	male
12	23.1	male
13	33.3	male

Figure 6.1 Part of a data file showing ages (highlighted) of male and female subjects

First, we confirm that the data come from normal distributions. The procedure for carrying this out is not shown here as it appears in Chapter 4.

It is also useful to plot the data. If we wish to plot the ages of each sex with error bars representing the standard error of the mean, first we make the selection shown in Figure 6.2.

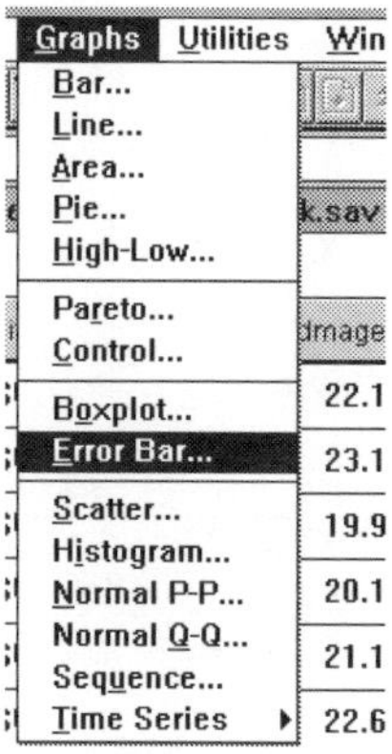

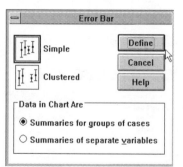

Figure 6.2 Selecting Error Bar in Graphs

Then press **Define** in the **Error Bar** box (Figure 6.3).

Figure 6.3 The Error Bar box

Make the appropriate choices in the dialogue box (Figure 6.4).

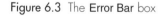

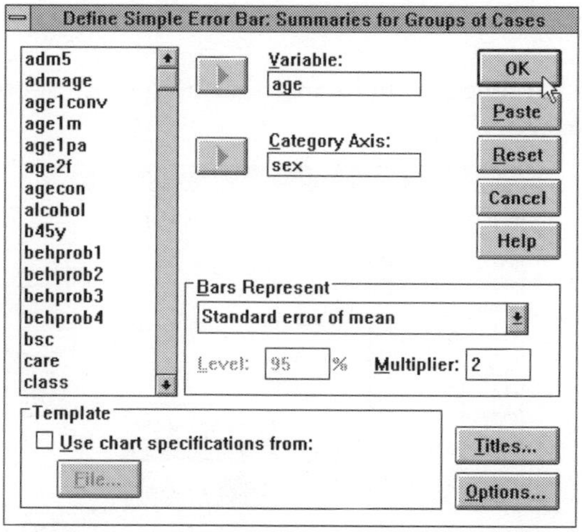

Figure 6.4 The Define Simple Error Bar: Summaries for Groups of Cases box

When **OK** is clicked, the required plot appears in the **Carousel**, as shown in Figure 6.5.

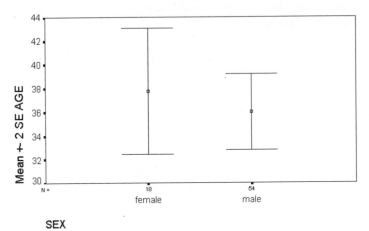

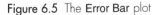

Figure 6.5 The **Error Bar** plot

The independent (unrelated) samples *t*-test procedure is chosen as shown in Figure 6.6.

Figure 6.6 Selecting the independent samples *t*-test

The appropriate variable selections are made in the corresponding dialogue box, as shown in Figure 6.7.

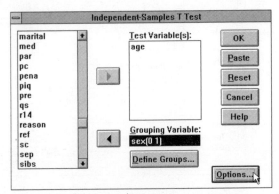

Figure 6.7 The **Independent-Samples T Test** box

(If a confidence interval other than 95% for the difference between the means is required, click on Options and make the necessary alteration.) Clicking on OK then gives the required results in the Output (Figure 6.8).

```
t-tests for Independent Samples of SEX

                              Number
Variable                     of Cases        Mean         SD    SE of Mean

AGE

fema                            18         37.7723      11.295     2.662
male                            54         36.0361      11.754     1.600


          Mean Difference = 1.7362

          Levene's Test for Equality of Variances: F= .221   P= .640


          t-test for Equality of Means                              95%
Variances   t-value      df     2-Tail Sig    SE of Diff       CI for Diff

Equal         .55        70        .586         3.169       (-4.585, 8.057)
Unequal       .56      30.23       .580         3.106       (-4.605, 8.077)
```

Figure 6.8 Output screen showing the results of an independent samples *t*-test

From the upper table in Figure 6.8 we can see that for the 18 female subjects, the mean age is 37.7723 years, with a standard deviation of 11.295 years and a standard error of the mean of 2.662 years. The corresponding figures for the 54 male subjects are 36.0361 years, 11.754 years and 1.600 years, respectively. Under this table we are told that the mean difference between the two groups is 1.7362 years.

The program automatically checks if the variances of the two groups are significantly different, using Levene's test. If the variances are *not* significantly different (using the F distribution) then the value of the probability adjacent to the value of F is greater than the significance level (commonly 5%, that is, 0.05). This is the case here, as shown in the highlighted output area in Figure 6.9.Therefore, in this case,

```
          Mean Difference = 1.7362

          Levene's Test for Equality of Variances: F= .221   P= .640
```

Figure 6.9 Part of the output screen of Figure 6.8 with Levene's test for equality of variances highlighted

the appropriate results are those in the upper row of the lower table of Figure 6.8 (Equal Variances), highlighted in Figure 6.10.

```
          Levene's Test for Equality of Variances: F= .221   P= .640


          t-test for Equality of Means                              95%
Variances   t-value      df     2-Tail Sig    SE of Diff       CI for Diff

Equal         .55        70        .586         3.169       (-4.585, 8.057)
Unequal       .56      30.23       .580         3.106       (-4.605, 8.077)
```

Figure 6.10 Part of the output screen of Figure 6.8 with the **Equal Variances** row of results highlighted

From this row we can see that the value of *t* is 0.55, which, with 70 degrees of freedom, corresponds to $P = 0.586$ (two-tailed), which is clearly not significant. Hence the ages of the male and female subjects are not significantly different. The 95% confidence interval for the difference between their ages is –4.585 to 8.057 years; this confidence interval includes the value zero, which is consistent with the finding that the ages of the two groups are not significantly different at the 5% level of significance. These findings are also consistent with the initial plot shown in Figure 6.5.

If Levineís test had shown that the variances were significantly different, then the second row (Unequal Variances) in Figure 6.10 would have been used instead.

Paired samples *t*-test

This procedure tests the null hypothesis that two population means are equal when the observations for the two groups can be paired in some way. For example, cases may consist of patients observed before and after an intervention, thereby giving rise to pairs of data. Pairing (a repeated measures or within-subjects design) is used to make the two groups as similar as possible, allowing differences observed between the two groups to be attributed more readily to the variable of interest.

Figure 6.11 shows the diastolic blood pressures of 12 men before and after a particular treatment.

1:before		78
	before	after
1	78	76
2	86	80
3	84	86
4	82	80
5	94	88
6	80	78
7	86	78
8	76	78
9	92	88
10	88	84
11	86	80
12	80	80

Figure 6.11 Part of a data file showing diastolic blood pressures of 12 male subjects before and after a certain treatment

Before running the paired samples *t*-test procedure, it is useful to plot the paired data as a scatterplot (scatter diagram or dot graph) by making the selection shown in Figures 6.12.

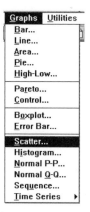

Figure 6.12 Selecting Scatter in Graphs

In the Scatterplot box choose the default Simple type of scatter diagram, and click Define (Figure 6.13).

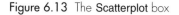

Figure 6.13 The Scatterplot box

In the next dialogue box select the two paired variables (Figure 6.14).

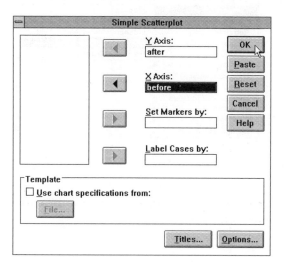

Figure 6.14 The Simple Scatterplot box

When OK is clicked, the required plot appears in the Carousel, as shown in Figure 6.15.

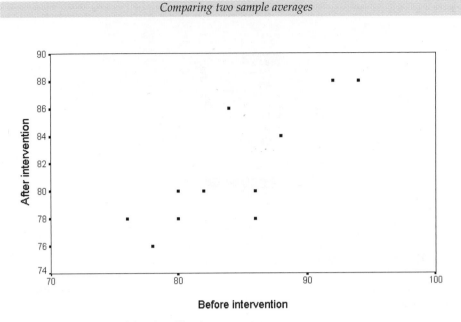

Figure 6.15 Scatterplot of the data file of Figure 6.11

With paired data, scatterplots allow anomalies in the data set to be checked for. In this case there are clearly no obvious outliers.

The paired (related) samples *t*-test procedure is chosen as shown in Figure 6.16.

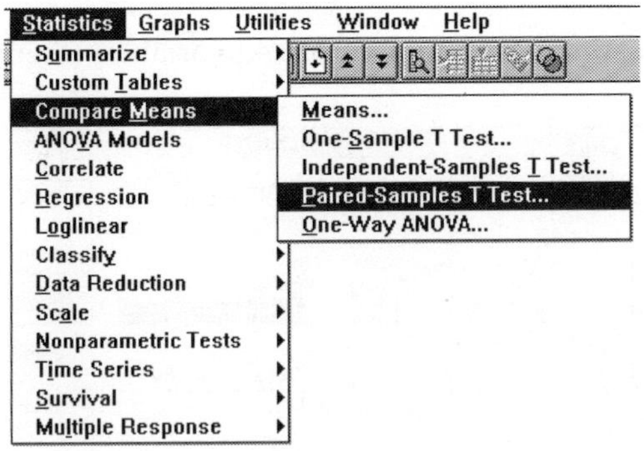

Figure 6.16 Selecting the paired samples *t*-test

The appropriate paired variable selection is made in the corresponding dialogue box, as shown in Figure 6.17.

```
t-tests for Paired Samples

               Number of           2-tail
Variable         pairs      Corr   Sig         Mean        SD      SE of Mean

AFTER    After intervention                   81.3333     4.119      1.189
                  12        .805   .002
BEFORE   Before intervention                  84.3333     5.449      1.573


         Paired Differences
   Mean          SD    SE of Mean         t-value         df      2-tail Sig

 -3.0000       3.247      .937            -3.20           11         .008
 95% CI (-5.063, -.937)
```

Figure 6.17 The **Paired-Samples *T* Test** box

(If a confidence interval other than 95% for the difference between the means is required, click on **Options** and make the necessary alteration.) Clicking on **OK** then gives the required results in the **Output** (Figure 6.18).

```
t-tests for Paired Samples

               Number of           2-tail
Variable         pairs      Corr   Sig         Mean        SD      SE of Mean

AFTER    After intervention                   81.3333     4.119      1.189
                  12        .805   .002
BEFORE   Before intervention                  84.3333     5.449      1.573


         Paired Differences
   Mean          SD    SE of Mean         t-value         df      2-tail Sig

 -3.0000       3.247      .937            -3.20           11         .008
 95% CI (-5.063, -.937)
```

Figure 6.18 Output screen showing the results of a paired samples *t*-test

From the upper part of Figure 6.18 we can see that the mean diastolic blood pressure after the intervention is 81.3333 mm Hg (millimetres of mercury), with a standard deviation of 4.119 mm Hg, while before the intervention the corresponding figures are 84.3333 and 5.449 mm Hg, respectively. The correlation coefficient (see Chapter 9) for the 12 pairs of observations is 0.805 (with an associated two-tailed significance value of 0.002). From the lower part of Figure 6.18 we can see that the mean difference between the two groups is −3.0000 mm Hg (that is, the diastolic blood pressure is on average 3 mm Hg *lower* after the intervention), with a standard deviation of 3.247 mm Hg. The value of *t* is −3.20, which, with 11 degrees of freedom, corresponds to $P = 0.008$ (two-tailed), which is clearly significant. Hence the diastolic blood pressure after the intervention is significantly lower than that before the intervention ($P = 0.008$). The 95% confidence interval for the difference is −5.063 to −0.937 mm Hg; this confidence interval does not include the value zero, which is consistent with the finding that the ages of the two groups are significantly different at the 5% level of significance.

NONPARAMETRIC TESTS

For data that do not fulfill the criteria for using parametric tests, SPSS offers non-parametric tests. As mentioned earlier in this book , note that nonparametric tests should not be used in preference if the data do fulfill the criteria for using parametric tests, since the nonparametric tests are less powerful, in a statistical sense, than their nonparametric equivalents.

Independent samples

The Mann–Whitney U test is an alternative to the independent samples t-test, in which the actual data values are replaced by ranks for the calculations.

Let us return again to the example of wishing to test the null hypothesis, at the 5% level of significance, that there is no difference between the population mean ages of the males and females in the data file shown in Figure 6.1. This time, suppose test of normality show that the data are not from normal distributions. Once again, we plot the data (Figure 6.5).

The Mann–Whitney U test is chosen as shown in Figure 6.19.

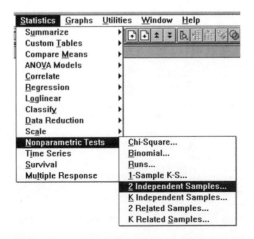

Figure 6.19 Selecting Nonparametric Tests: Two Independent Samples

The appropriate variable selections are made in the corresponding dialogue box, as shown in Figure 6.20.

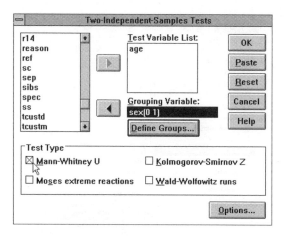

Figure 6.20 The Two-Independent-Samples Tests box

Clicking on **OK** then gives the required results in the Output (Figure 6.21).

```
- - - - - Mann-Whitney U - Wilcoxon Rank Sum W Test

        AGE
   by SEX


      Mean Rank    Cases

        39.67         18   SEX = 0   female
        35.44         54   SEX = 1   male
                      --
                      72   Total

                                   Corrected for ties
              U           W          Z        2-Tailed P
          429.0        714.0      -.7413        .4585
```

Figure 6.21 Output screen showing the results of a Mann–Whitney U test

From this **Output** we can see that there is no significant difference between the ages of the male and female subjects according to this nonparametric test ($P = 0.4585$ (two-tailed)).

Paired (related) samples

Let us return again to the example of testing the null hypothesis that there is no difference between the diastolic blood pressures of 12 men before and after a particular treatment, for the dataset shown in Figure 6.11. The scatterplot for these data has already been plotted (Figure 6.15).

The nonparametric tests for paired (two related) samples are selected as shown in Figure 6.22.

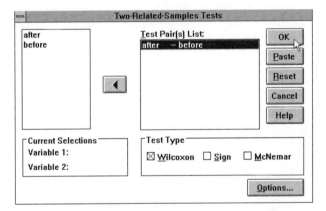

Figure 6.22 Selecting the nonparametric tests for paired (two related) samples

The appropriate paired variable selection is made in the corresponding dialogue box, as shown in Figure 6.23.

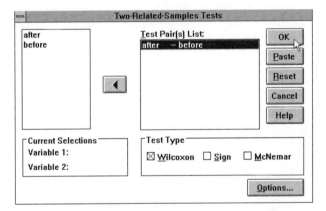

Figure 6.23 The Two-Related-Samples Tests box

Three nonparametric tests are offered, as follows.

- The Wilcoxon matched-pairs test makes no assumptions about the shapes of the distribution of the two variables. The absolute values of the differences between the two variables are calculated for each case and ranked from smallest to largest. The test statistic is based on the sums of ranks for negative and positive differences. It is more powerful, statistically, than the Sign test.
- The Sign test is based on the directions of the differences between two variables.
- McNemar's test is used to determine changes in proportions for related samples. It is often used for 'before and after' experimental designs when the dependent variable is dichotomous.

Since our data are not dichotomous, we have a choice between the first two, and will choose the more powerful test, namely the Wilcoxon matched-pairs test. This has been chosen in Figure 6.23. Clicking on OK then gives the required results in the Output (Figure 6.24).

```
 - - - - - Wilcoxon Matched-Pairs Signed-Ranks Test

        AFTER      After intervention
  with BEFORE      Before intervention


      Mean Rank    Cases

          3.00         2   - Ranks (BEFORE LT AFTER)
          6.67         9   + Ranks (BEFORE GT AFTER)
                       1     Ties  (BEFORE EQ AFTER)
                      --
                      12     Total

          Z =   -2.4006            2-Tailed P =   .0164
```

Figure 6.24 Output screen showing the results of a Wilcoxon matched-pairs test

From this **Output** we see that, according to this nonparametric test, the diastolic blood pressure after the intervention is significantly lower than that before the intervention ($P = 0.0164$ (two-tailed)).

7 CONTINGENCY TABLES

DEFINITION

A contingency table, referred to as a crosstabulation in SPSS, is a table with a cell for every combination of values of two or more variables. The table shows the number of cases with each specific combination of values.

A contingency table with r rows and c columns is referred to as a $r \times c$ contingency table. Note that in counting the number of rows and columns variable labels and marginal totals are not taken into account. For example, the core of a hypothetical 4 $\times$ 2 contingency table is shown in Figure 7.1.

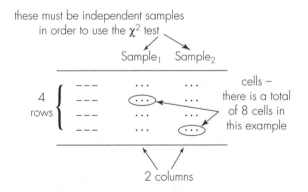

Figure 7.1 The core structure of a 4 × 2 contingency table. Based on Puri BK and Tyrer P (1992) *Sciences Basic to Psychiatry*, with permission from Churchill Livingstone, Edinburgh

Figure 7.1 can be expanded by adding in the marginal totals (Figure 7.2); this does not alter the number of rows (four) or number of columns (two).

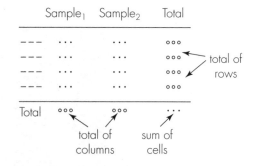

Figure 7.2 A 4 × 2 contingency table with added marginal totals. Based on Puri BK and Tyrer P (1992) *Sciences Basic to Psychiatry*, with permission from Churchill Livingstone, Edinburgh

CONDITIONS

In this chapter we describe how to compare independent unrelated categorical data presented in the form of contingency tables. The general conditions for using the tests described are:

- the data are categorical, that is, either nominal (qualitative) or ordinal (assigned to ordered categories)
- the actual values of the data, that is, their frequencies, should be used in the contingency tables; proportions, including percentages, should not be used
- the variables should be independent and unrelated
- the parent populations of the samples compared do not have to have any particular distribution; the tests described are non-parametric.

Further conditions for the use of the chi-square test are given in the next section.

CHI-SQUARE TEST

The chi-square (χ^2) test is used to test the hypothesis that the row and column variables of a contingency table are independent.

The number of degrees of freedom of a contingency table is given by (number of rows − 1) × (number of columns − 1). So, a 2 × 2 table has one degree of freedom.

In addition to the general conditions given above, the following criteria should be fulfilled for the chi-square test to be valid for a contingency table with more than one degree of freedom:

- each expected value 1
- in at least 80% of cases, expected value greater than 5.

SPSS automatically notes whether or not these criteria are fulfilled when using the chi-square test.

Figure 7.3 shows part of a data file from a study on dyslexia, with dyslexic status (normal control or dyslexic) and handedness group (right consistent, mixed preference or left consistent) highlighted. We shall test the null hypothesis that these two variables are independent using the chi-square test.

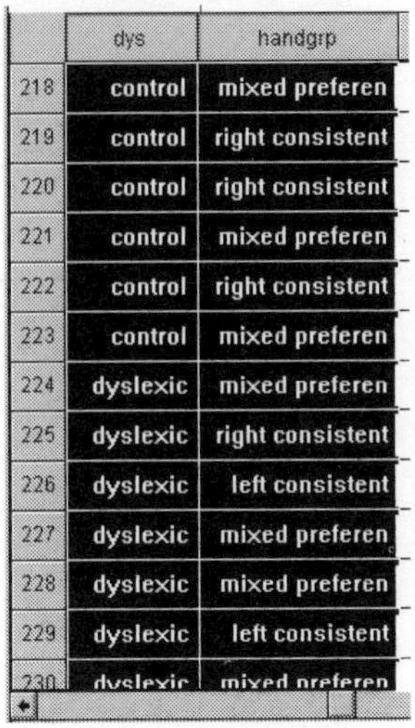

	dys	handgrp
218	control	mixed preferen
219	control	right consistent
220	control	right consistent
221	control	mixed preferen
222	control	right consistent
223	control	mixed preferen
224	dyslexic	mixed preferen
225	dyslexic	right consistent
226	dyslexic	left consistent
227	dyslexic	mixed preferen
228	dyslexic	mixed preferen
229	dyslexic	left consistent
230	dyslexic	mixed preferen

Figure 7.3 Part of a data file from a study on dyslexia, with dyslexic status (dys) and handedness group (handgrp) highlighted

Crosstabs (for crosstabulation) is selected, as shown in Figure 7.4.

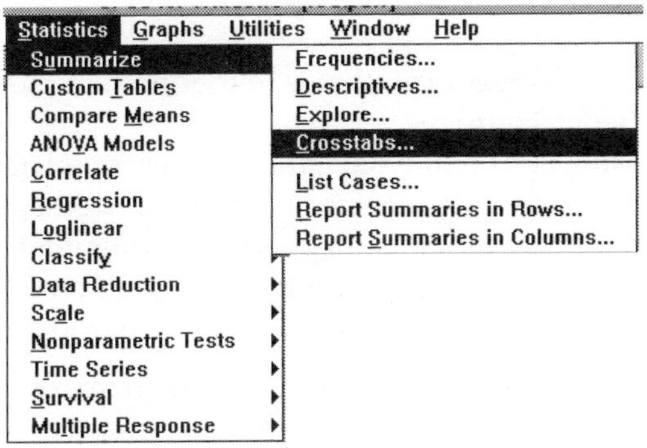

Statistics	Graphs	Utilities	Window	Help
Summarize		Frequencies...		
Custom Tables		Descriptives...		
Compare Means		Explore...		
ANOVA Models		Crosstabs...		
Correlate				
Regression		List Cases...		
Loglinear		Report Summaries in Rows...		
Classify		Report Summaries in Columns...		
Data Reduction ▶				
Scale ▶				
Nonparametric Tests ▶				
Time Series ▶				
Survival ▶				
Multiple Response ▶				

Figure 7.4 Selecting Crosstabs

In the resulting Crosstabs box the required variables are selected, as shown in Figure 7.5.

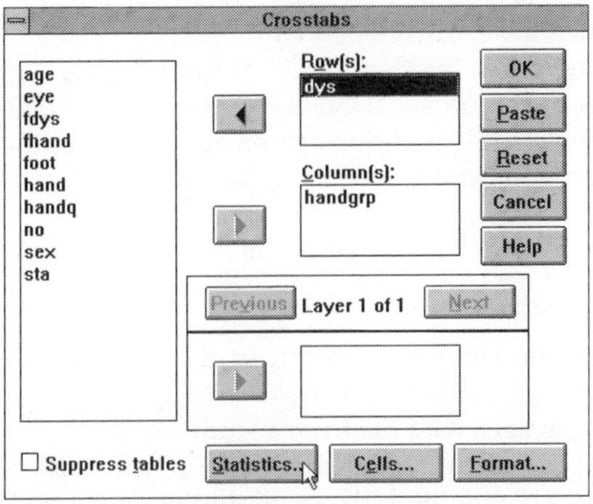

Crosstabs

age
eye
fdys
fhand
foot
hand
handq
no
sex
sta

Row(s):
dys

Column(s):
handgrp

Previous Layer 1 of 1 Next

OK
Paste
Reset
Cancel
Help

☐ Suppress tables   Statistics...   Cells...   Format...

Figure 7.5 The Crosstabs box

Click on Statistics... and in the resulting Crosstabs: Statistics box select Chi-square (Figure 7.6).

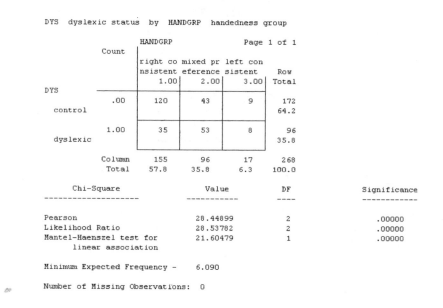

Figure 7.6 The Crosstabs: Statistics box

Click on Continue to return to the Crosstabs box. Clicking on OK then takes you to the Output screen with the results of the chi-square analysis, shown in Figure 7.7.

```
DYS   dyslexic status  by  HANDGRP  handedness group

                      HANDGRP                 Page 1 of 1
              Count
                      right co mixed pr left con
                      nsistent eference sistent      Row
                         1.00|    2.00|    3.00| Total
DYS           _____
                .00     120      43        9       172
    control                                        64.2

               1.00     35       53        8        96
    dyslexic                                        35.8

             Column    155      96        17       268
             Total     57.8     35.8      6.3     100.0

      Chi-Square                  Value         DF      Significance
--------------------          -----------      ----    ------------

Pearson                        28.44899         2         .00000
Likelihood Ratio               28.53782         2         .00000
Mantel-Haenszel test for       21.60479         1         .00000
    linear association

Minimum Expected Frequency -    6.090

Number of Missing Observations:  0
```

Figure 7.7 Output screen showing the results of a chi-square test

From this Output we can see that the value of chi-square (appearing in the row labelled Pearson) is 28.44899, with 2 degrees of freedom (because this is a 2×3 table). This is seen to be highly significant (significance given as .00000, that is, less than 0.000 005) and so the null hypothesis that the variables, dyslexia and handedness, are independent can be rejected. From the table in Figure 7.7 we can see that this result is caused by an excess of mixed handedness preference in the dyslexic group. This can be made easier to assess if the frequency values which would be expected under the null hypothesis are included in the table. This option is chosen by clicking Cells... in the Crosstabs box, as shown in Figure 7.8.

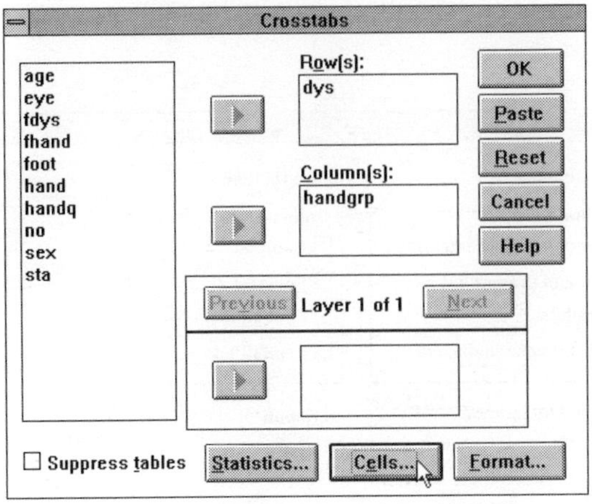

Figure 7.8 Selecting **Cells...** in the **Crosstabs** box

In the resulting box select **Expected** as shown in Figure 7.9.

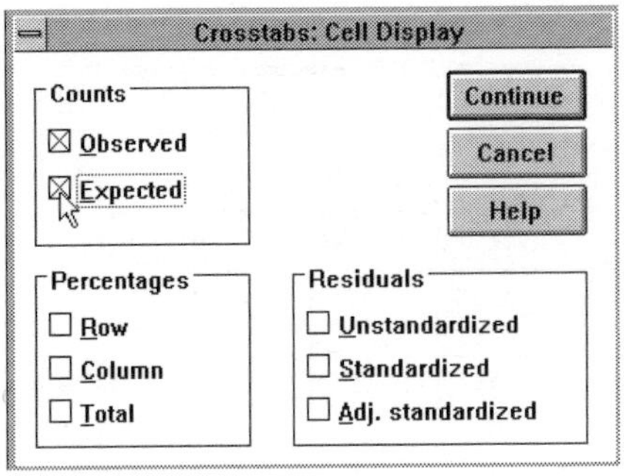

Figure 7.9 The **Crosstabs: Cell Display** box

Click on **Continue** to return to the **Crosstabs** box. Clicking on **OK** takes you to the Output screen with the results of the chi-square analysis, but this time the table appears as shown in Figure 7.10.

		HANDGRP		Page 1 of 1	
	Count Exp Val	right co nsistent 1.00	mixed pr eference 2.00	left con sistent 3.00	Row Total
DYS					
control	.00	120 99.5	43 61.6	9 10.9	172 64.2%
dyslexic	1.00	35 55.5	53 34.4	8 6.1	96 35.8%
	Column Total	155 57.8%	96 35.8%	17 6.3%	268 100.0%

Figure 7.10 Contingency table in **Output** including both observed and expected frequencies

In each cell the upper figure is the actual observed count, while the lower figure is the frequency expected under the null hypothesis.

FISHER'S EXACT TEST

Fisher's exact probability test is a test for independence in a 2×2 table. It determines the exact probability of obtaining the observed result or one more extreme, if the two variables are independent and the marginal totals are fixed.

SPSS automatically checks if it is dealing with a 2×2 table with any expected value less than five, or a total sample size of 20 or less, in which case it then proceeds with this test. For example, in the output shown in Figure 7.11, SPSS has determined that, for the contingency table shown, two (50%) out of four of the cells has an expected value of less than five. Therefore Fisher's exact probability test has automatically been carried out, from which it can be seen that the probability of obtaining the observed result or one more extreme is 0.17436 (two-tailed). Thus the null hypothesis that the two groups studied are independent cannot be rejected.

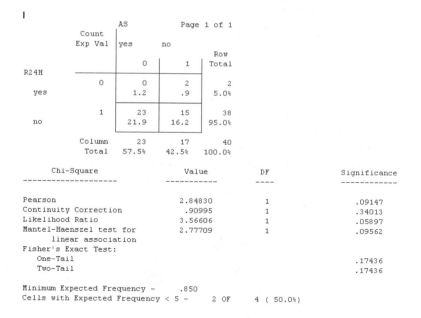

```
                  AS              Page 1 of 1
            Count
            Exp Val   yes      no
                                        Row
                        0        1      Total
      R24H
                0       0        2         2
      yes              1.2      .9       5.0%

                1       23       15       38
      no              21.9     16.2     95.0%

            Column     23       17       40
            Total    57.5%    42.5%    100.0%


        Chi-Square               Value      DF      Significance
      --------------------       -------    ----    ------------

      Pearson                   2.84830      1        .09147
      Continuity Correction      .90995      1        .34013
      Likelihood Ratio          3.56606      1        .05897
      Mantel-Haenszel test for  2.77709      1        .09562
         linear association
      Fisher's Exact Test:
         One-Tail                                     .17436
         Two-Tail                                     .17436

      Minimum Expected Frequency -    .850
      Cells with Expected Frequency < 5 -    2 OF    4 ( 50.0%)
```

Figure 7.11 Output screen showing the results of an analysis using Fisher's exact test

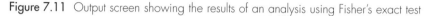

ENTERING A CONTINGENCY TABLE

In the above examples, the contingency tables shown in the Output screens have been produced by SPSS on the basis of the raw data in the corresponding data files. Sometimes, however, you may wish to analyze a completed contingency table without having to enter all its raw data. Furthermore, sometimes the raw data may not be available. For example, you may wish to check the results of a published contingency table, such as that shown in Table 7.1, which shows the orientation (clockwise or anticlockwise) of the parietal scalp hair whorl in two groups of people (patients with schizophrenia and normal controls).

Table 7.1 Parietal hair whorl orientation in schizophrenia. (From Puri, BK *et al.* (1995) Parietal scalp hair whorl patterns in schizophrenia. *Biological Psychiatry*, **37**, 278–9.)

	Clockwise	Anticlockwise
Schizophrenic patients	114	12
($n = 126$)	(90.5%)	(9.5%)
Normal controls	1629	261
$n = 890$	(86.2%)	(13.8%)

These data can be entered directly as a data file in the form shown in Figure 7.12.

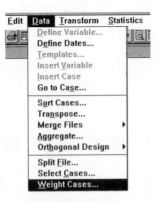

	subjects	whorl	count	var
1	schizophrenic	clockwise	114	
2	schizophrenic	anticlockwise	12	
3	normal control	clockwise	1629	
4	normal control	anticlockwise	261	
5				

Figure 7.12 Entering the data of the contingency table shown in Table 7.1 directly into a data file

The first two variables in this data file represent the rows and columns of the contingency table, while the third variable represents the frequencies (count) for each corresponding cell of the table. In order that SPSS treats the the last column (count) as one that contains the cell frequencies, the **Weight Cases** box is selected, as shown in Figure 7.13.

```
Edit  Data  Transform  Statistics
      Define Variable...
      Define Dates...
      Templates...
      Insert Variable
      Insert Case
      Go to Case...

      Sort Cases...
      Transpose...
      Merge Files        ▶
      Aggregate...
      Orthogonal Design  ▶

      Split File...
      Select Cases...
      Weight Cases...
```

Figure 7.13 Selecting the **Weight Cases** box

In the **Weight Cases** box, make the selection shown in Figure 7.14, so informing SPSS that there is a frequency variable (count) by which cases should be weighted.

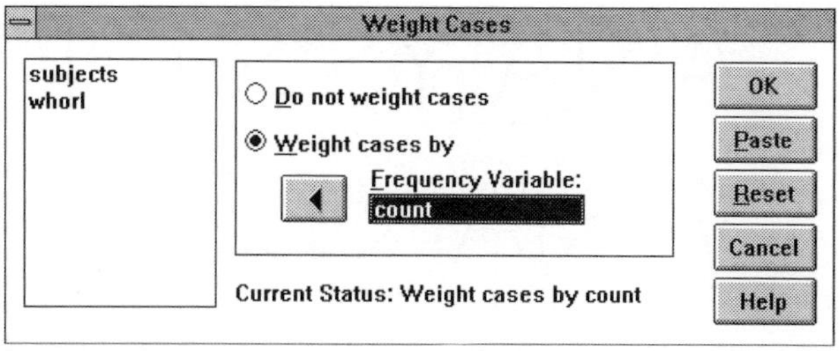

Figure 7.14 The Weight Cases box

Click OK and then proceed to carry out the analysis as described earlier in this chapter. The resulting Output is shown in Figure 7.15.

```
SUBJECTS  by  WHORL

                     WHORL          Page 1 of 1
             Count
             Exp Val  clockwis anticloc
                      e        kwise       Row
                          1         2      Total
SUBJECTS     ────────
             1          114       12        126
schizophrenic          108.9     17.1       6.3%

             2          1629      261       1890
normal control         1634.1    255.9      93.8%

          Column        1743      273       2016
          Total         86.5%     13.5%     100.0%

      Chi-Square                Value        DF        Significance
----------------------        ----------    ----      ------------

Pearson                        1.85314        1          .17342
Continuity Correction          1.50517        1          .21988
Likelihood Ratio               2.02445        1          .15478
Mantel-Haenszel test for       1.85223        1          .17352
   linear association

Minimum Expected Frequency -    17.063


Number of Missing Observations:   0
```

Figure 7.15 Output based on the data of Table 7.1

From this Output it can be seen that the value of χ^2 for Table 7.1 is 1.85314. On one degree of freedom, this is not significant ($P = 0.17342$), and so we must accept the null hypothesis that there is no statistically significant difference between the two groups.

8 ANALYSIS OF VARIANCE

Analysis of variance, usually abbreviated to ANOVA, is a method of testing the null hypothesis that several group means are equal in the population, by comparing the sample variance estimated from the group means to that estimated within the groups. In this chapter the application of the following three types of ANOVA using SPSS are described:

one-way ANOVA
simple factorial ANOVA
repeated measures ANOVA.

ONE-WAY ANOVA

This procedure tests the null hypothesis that the data are a sample from a population in which the mean of a test variable is equal in several independent groups of cases defined by a single grouping variable. The 'one-way' in its name comes from the fact that the cases are allocated to the independent groups on the basis of values for that one test variable. There are no repeated measures.

PARAMETRIC TEST

The parametric test is a generalization of the independent samples t-test (see Chapter 6). Indeed, when using one-way ANOVA to compare two groups, the results obtained are the same as when an independent samples t-test is carried out. It is important not to substitute the carrying out of multiple t-tests to compare each pair of sample means for an ANOVA; the former procedure would greatly increase the chance that a significant difference will falsely be found.

Assumptions

The following assumptions are made.

- The data are measured on a ratio or interval scale. If the data are ordinal, then a non-parametric test should be carried out instead, as described below.
- Each group is an independent random sample. If the data contain repeated measures, then a repeated measures ANOVA, described later in this chapter, should be used instead.

- Each group comes from a normally distributed population. This assumption should be checked as described in Chapter 4. If the data are not normal, then it may be possible to make them so by transformation (for example taking square roots, reciprocals or logarithms). If this does not work, then a non-parametric ANOVA can be used instead, as described later in this chapter.
- The population variances are equal. This assumption can be checked by carrying out a test of homogeneity of variance (using the Levene test of equality of variance). Alternatively, since the one-way ANOVA is fairly robust to small deviations from this assumption, a box-plot can be produced, as described in Chapter 4, and the spread of the groups can thereby be checked. If there is marked heterogeneity of variance, then a non-parametric ANOVA can be used instead, as described later in this chapter.

Procedure

Table 8.1 shows the plasticity, in arbitrary units, of a group of five independent random samples of each of three different materials, A, B and C. The question to be answered is whether the plasticities of the materials differ.

Table 8.1 Plasticity of three materials A to C. Based on Puri, BK (1996) *Statistics for the Health Sciences*, with permission from WB Saunders, London

A	13	14	15	14	16
B	16	13	12	11	13
C	14	10	11	13	15

The data have been entered into a data file, as shown in Figure 8.1.

	plasticy	material
1	13	A
2	14	A
3	15	A
4	14	A
5	16	A
6	16	B
7	13	B
8	12	B
9	11	B
10	13	B
11	14	C
12	10	C
13	11	C
14	13	C
15	15	C

[Figure 8.1 The data of Table 8.1 in a data file

The one-way ANOVA procedure is selected as shown in Figure 8.2.

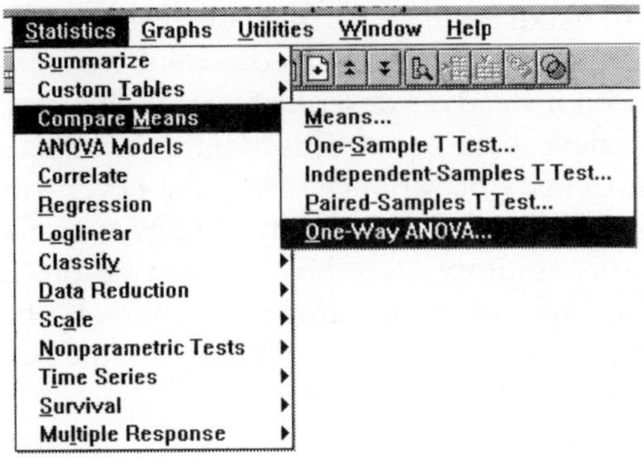

Figure 8.2 Selecting **One-way ANOVA**

The one-way ANOVA box is completed, as shown in Figure 8.3 (the grouping factor, material, has a range from 1 to 3, corresponding to materials A to C, respectively).

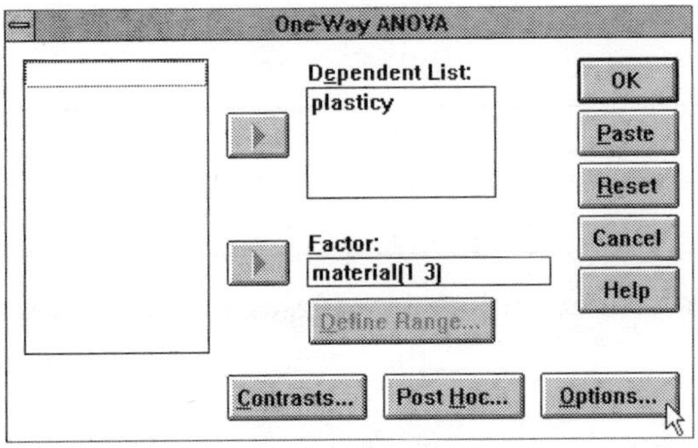

Figure 8.3 The **One-way ANOVA** box

Click the **Options...** button to obtain the **One-way ANOVA: Options** box (see Figure 8.4), in which **Descriptive** can be selected, to give the descriptive statistics for the data, and **Homogeneity-of-variance** can be selected to carry out the Levine test for homogeneity of variances.

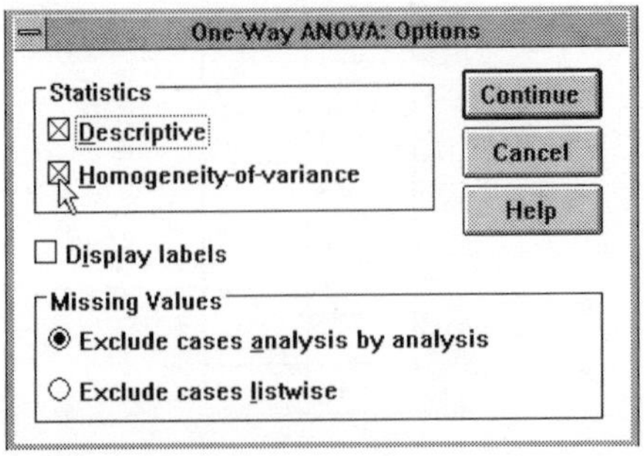

Figure 8.4 The **One-way ANOVA**: Options box

Click Continue to return to the One-way ANOVA box, and then click OK. The Output has three components, in the following order:

- the ANOVA
- descriptive statistics
- the Levine test for homogeneity of variances.

Figure 8.5 shows the result of the Levine test for homogeneity of variances, with the two-tailed significance probability highlighted.

```
         Levene Test for Homogeneity of Variances

            Statistic    df1    df2    2-tail Sig.
               .8673       2     12        .445
```

Figure 8.5 Output from **One-way ANOVA**: the Levine test for homogeneity of variances (with the two-tailed significance probability highlighted)

It can be seen that the value of this probability is 0.445, which means that the variances can be taken as not being significantly different.

Figure 8.6 shows the result of the ANOVA, with the value of F (F Ratio) and its corresponding probability (F Prob.) highlighted.

```
              - - - - - O N E W A Y - - - - -

        Variable  PLASTICY   plasticity
     By Variable  MATERIAL

                           Analysis of Variance

                              Sum of       Mean        F      F
            Source      D.F.  Squares      Squares    Ratio  Prob.

    Between Groups        2    8.9333      4.4667     1.4725  .2680
    Within Groups        12   36.4000      3.0333
    Total                14   45.3333
```

Figure 8.6 Output from **One-way ANOVA** the result of the ANOVA (with the value of F and its corresponding probability highlighted)

It can be seen that the value of this probability is 0.2680, which means that the null hypothesis that the population means are not different cannot be rejected.

Figure 8.7 shows the descriptive statistics.

Group	Count	Mean	Standard Deviation	Standard Error	95 Pct Conf Int for Mean		
Grp 1	5	14.4000	1.1402	.5099	12.9843	TO	15.8157
Grp 2	5	13.0000	1.8708	.8367	10.6771	TO	15.3229
Grp 3	5	12.6000	2.0736	.9274	10.0253	TO	15.1747
Total	15	13.3333	1.7995	.4646	12.3368	TO	14.3298

GROUP	MINIMUM	MAXIMUM
Grp 1	13.0000	16.0000
Grp 2	11.0000	16.0000
Grp 3	10.0000	15.0000

Figure 8.7 Output from **One-way ANOVA**: the descriptive statistics

Multiple comparisons

While a one-way ANOVA resulting in a statistically significant value of F allows the null hypothesis (that the population means are equal) to be rejected, it does not indicate which means are significantly different. In order to determine this, a multiple comparisons procedure needs to be carried out, either unplanned after it is known that the value of F is statistically significant (*post hoc*) or planned before the value of F is determined (*a priori*). As mentioned above, multiple t-tests comparing each pair of sample means should not be carried out, as this would greatly increase the chance that a significant difference will falsely be found.

A multiple comparison test can be chosen by clicking the **Post Hoc...** button in the **One-Way ANOVA** box (see Figure 8.3) and selecting the appropriate test from the options available shown in Figure 8.8.

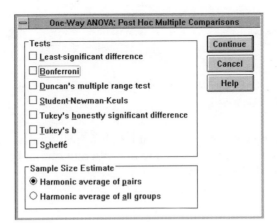

Figure 8.8 The **One-way ANOVA: Post Hoc Multiple Comparisons** box

For example, suppose the data in Table 8.1 and Figure 8.1 appeared as in Figure 8.9. (Compared with the data in Figure 8.1, material A has higher plasticity ratings.)

	plasticy	material
1	18	A
2	19	A
3	20	A
4	19	A
5	21	A
6	16	B
7	13	B
8	12	B
9	11	B
10	13	B
11	14	C
12	10	C
13	11	C
14	13	C
15	15	C

Figure 8.9 The data of Figure 8.1 modified (higher plasticity ratings for material A)

This time, running a one-way ANOVA results in the Output shown in Figure 8.10.

```
- - - - -  O N E W A Y  - - - - -


    Variable  PLASTICY   plasticity
  By Variable  MATERIAL

                          Analysis of Variance


                          Sum of        Mean          F     F
         Source     D.F.  Squares       Squares      Ratio  Prob.

Between Groups       2    145.6000      72.8000      24.0000 .0001
Within Groups       12     36.4000       3.0333
Total               14    182.0000
```

Figure 8.10 Output from **One-way ANOVA** for the data in Figure 8.9 (the value of F and its corresponding probability are highlighted)

The null hypothesis can be rejected ($P = 0.0001$). In order to determine which group means differ significantly from each other, we now examine the results of the multiple comparison procedure. In this case the Bonferroni test (which uses t-tests to carry out pairwise comparisons between the group means but takes into account the number of tests) has been selected, and part of the results are shown in Figure 8.11.

```
(*) Indicates significant differences which are shown in the lower triangle

                               G G G
                               r r r
                               p p p

                               3 2 1
          Mean        MATERIAL

         12.6000      Grp 3
         13.0000      Grp 2
         19.4000      Grp 1       * *

Homogeneous Subsets (highest and lowest means are not significantly different)

Subset 1

Group        Grp 3           Grp 2

Mean         12.6000         13.0000
- - - - - - - - - - - - - -

Subset 2

Group        Grp 1

Mean         19.4000
- - - - - -
```

Figure 8.11 Part of the results of a Bonferroni test corresponding to the **Output** in Figure 8.10

From the upper part of Figure 8.11 it can be seen that group 1 (material A) differs significantly from groups 2 (B) and 3 (C). In the lower part of Figure 8.11 it can be seen that the groups have been subdivided into homogeneous subsets. Subset 1 consists of materials B and C which do not differ significantly from each other, while subset 2 contains material A alone.

NON-PARAMETRIC TESTS

A non-parametric ANOVA should be carried out if the data do not fulfill the criteria for the parametric test given above.

Kruskal–Wallis test

The Kruskal–Wallis test is a non-parametric alternative to the parametric test just described requires that the data be measured at least on an ordinal scale. The test statistic (H) is calculated in the same way as the Mann–Whitney test statistic (a non-parametric alternative to the independent samples *t*-test).

We shall illustrate the use of this test by applying it to the data shown in Table 8.1 and Figure 8.1. The procedure is selected as shown in Figure 8.12.

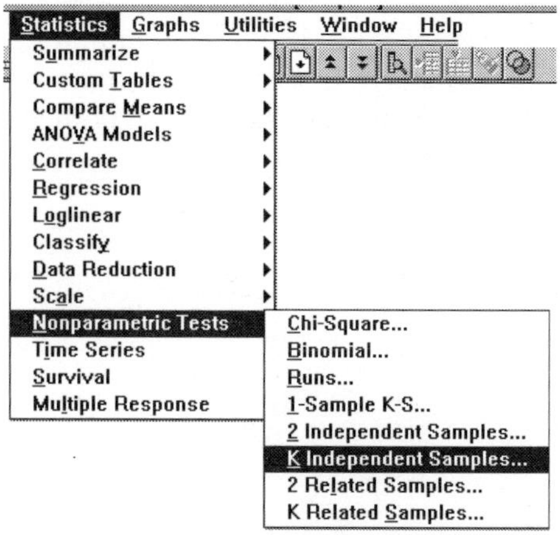

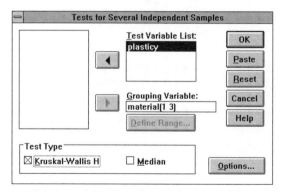

Figure 8.12 Selecting Nonparametric tests: K Independent Samples

The resulting box is filled in as shown in Figure 8.13.

Figure 8.13 The Tests for Several Independent Samples box

Click the Options... button to obtain the Options box (see Figure 8.14), in which Descriptive or Quartiles can be selected, to give the descriptive statistics for the data.

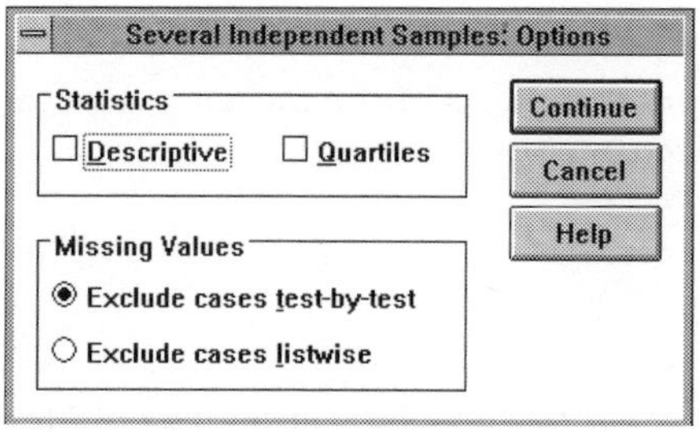

Figure 8.14 The Tests for Several Independent Samples: Options box

Click **Continue** to return to the **Tests for Several Independent Samples** box, and then click **OK**. From the **Output** (Figure 8.15), it can be seen that the required probability (corrected for ties) is 0.2428 (in this case similar to the parametric test probability of 0.2680 found above), which means that the null hypothesis that the population means are not different cannot be rejected.

```
 - - - - - Kruskal-Wallis 1-Way Anova

     PLASTICY   plasticity
  by MATERIAL


   Mean Rank    Cases

      10.70        5     MATERIAL = 1    A
       6.80        5     MATERIAL = 2    B
       6.50        5     MATERIAL = 3    C

                  --

                  15     Total

                                        Corrected for ties
   Chi-Square    D.F.  Significance   Chi-Square      D.F.  Significance
      2.7450        2        .2535       2.8309          2        .2428
```

Figure 8.15 Output from Kruskal–Wallis one-way ANOVA

Median test

This non-parametric procedure tests whether two or more samples are drawn from populations with the same median. It uses the chi-square statistic (see Chapter 7) and therefore should not be used if any cell has an expected frequency of less than one or if more than 20 per cent of cells have expected frequencies of less than five. It is carried out by selecting **Median** in the **Tests for Several Independent Samples** box (Figure 8.13) and clicking **OK**.

SIMPLE FACTORIAL ANOVA

Simple factorial ANOVA differs from one-way ANOVA in that it can handle several grouping variables (factors) simultaneously. The criteria that need to be fulfilled for using this test are otherwise essentially the same as those listed under Assumptions in the previous section on One-way ANOVA.

With more than one factor, two types of 'treatment' effects (in ANOVA terminology) can occur:

● main effects, which are the effects of the individual factors
● an interaction between factors; that is, the effects of the factors are mutually dependent.

Procedure

Figure 8.16 shows part of a data file which contains both the plasticity (in arbitrary units) and the method of measuring the plasticity (using one of five methods labelled 1 to 5) of three materials, A, B and C, for a total of 25 cases.

	plasticy	material	method
1	18	A	1
2	10	A	2
3	20	A	3
4	19	A	4
5	21	A	5
6	16	B	1
7	4	B	2
8	12	B	3
9	11	B	4
10	13	B	5
11	14	· C	1
12	11	C	2
13	11	C	3
14	13	C	4
15	15	C	5
16	16	A	1

Figure 8.16 Part of a data file showing both the plasticity and the method of measuring the plasticity (methods 1 to 5) of three materials, A, B and C for a total of 25 cases

The corresponding means and standard deviations are obtained by making the selection shown in Figure 8.17.

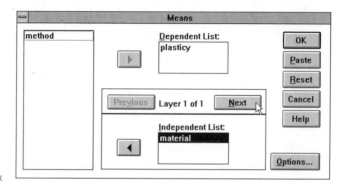

Statistics	Graphs	Utilities	Window	Help
Summarize				
Custom Tables				
Compare Means		Means...		
ANOVA Models		One-Sample T Test...		
Correlate		Independent-Samples T Test...		
Regression		Paired-Samples T Test...		
Loglinear		One-Way ANOVA...		
Classify				
Data Reduction				
Scale				
Nonparametric Tests				
Time Series				
Survival				
Multiple Response				

Figure 8.17 Selecting Compare Means: Means

In the Means box, plasticity is entered as the dependent variable in the Dependent List, and material in the Independent List, as shown in Figure 8.18.

Figure 8.18 The Means box

To enter the next layer of classification, click the Next button and in the resulting box enter the variable method, as shown in Figure 8.19.

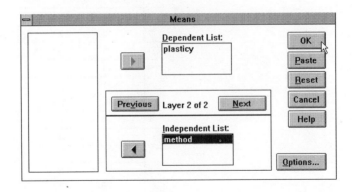

Figure 8.19 Entering layer 2 of 2 in the **Means** box

Click **OK** to obtain the **Output** shown in Figure 8.20. (Notice that a standard deviation is not given when the number of cases in a cell is one.)

```
 ↕                      - - Description of Subpopulations - -

  Summaries of      PLASTICY    plasticity
  By levels of      MATERIAL
                    METHOD                        )

  Variable          Value  Label              Mean    Std Dev    Cases

  For Entire Population                       13.1200   4.0755      25

  MATERIAL            1  A                    15.4286   6.2144       7
    METHOD            1                       17.0000   1.4142       2
    METHOD            2                        7.0000   4.2426       2
    METHOD            3                       20.0000      .         1
    METHOD            4                       19.0000      .         1
    METHOD            5                       21.0000      .         1

  MATERIAL            2  B                    11.7000   3.1287      10
    METHOD            1                       15.0000   1.4142       2
    METHOD            2                        7.5000   4.9497       2
    METHOD            3                       12.0000    .0000       2
    METHOD            4                       11.0000    .0000       2
    METHOD            5                       13.0000    .0000       2

  MATERIAL            3  C                    12.8750   1.7269       8
    METHOD            1                       14.0000      .         1
    METHOD            2                       11.0000      .         1
    METHOD            3                       11.0000    .0000       2
    METHOD            4                       13.0000    .0000       2
    METHOD            5                       15.0000    .0000       2

    Total Cases = 25
```

Figure 8.20 Output showing summary means and standard deviations of plasticity by levels of material and method

To obtain the means and standard deviations for the variable method, re-open the **Means** box and complete it as shown in Figure 8.21.

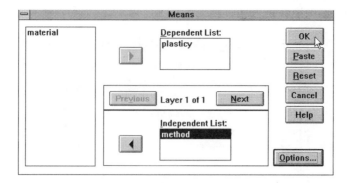

Figure 8.21 The **Means** box completed in order to obtain summary means and standard deviations for levels of the second independent variable (method) of Figures. 8.19 and 8.20

The resulting **Output** is shown in Figure 8.22.

```
                    - - Description of Subpopulations - -

Summaries of     PLASTICY     plasticity
By levels of     METHOD


Variable       Value  Label                    Mean    Std Dev   Cases

For Entire Population                         13.1200    4.0755     25

METHOD            1                           15.6000    1.6733      5
METHOD            2                            8.0000    3.6742      5
METHOD            3                           13.2000    3.8341      5
METHOD            4                           13.4000    3.2863      5
METHOD            5                           15.4000    3.2863      5

    Total Cases = 25
```

Figure 8.22 Output showing summary means and standard deviations of plasticity by method

To run a simple factorial ANOVA, make the selection shown in Figure 8.23.

Statistics	Graphs	Utilities	Window	Help

Summarize ▶
Custom Tables ▶
Compare Means ▶
ANOVA Models ▶   Simple Factorial...
Correlate   General Factorial...
Regression   Multivariate...
Loglinear   Repeated Measures...
Classify
Data Reduction ▶
Scale ▶
Nonparametric Tests ▶
Time Series ▶
Survival ▶
Multiple Response ▶

Figure 8.23 Selecting Simple Factorial ANOVA

Analysis of variance

The Simple Factorial ANOVA box is completed as shown in Figure 8.24 (the factor material has a range from 1 to 3, corresponding to materials A to C, respectively, while the factor method has a range from 1 to 5).

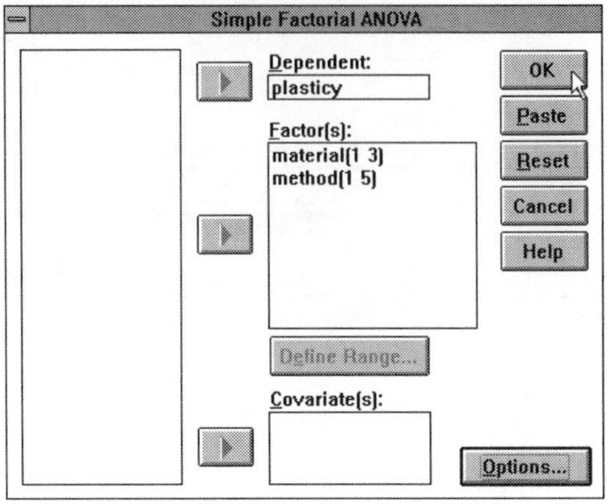

Figure 8.24 The **Simple Factorial ANOVA** box

Clicking **OK** leads to the **Output** shown in Figure 8.25, in which the relevant *F* ratios and their corresponding probabilities (Sig of F) have been highlighted.

```
          * * *  A N A L Y S I S   O F   V A R I A N C E  * * *

              PLASTICY plasticity
          by  MATERIAL
              METHOD

              UNIQUE sums of squares
              All effects entered simultaneously

                                  Sum of              Mean              Sig
          Source of Variation     Squares     DF      Square      F     of F

          Main Effects            250.035     6       41.672     8.962   .002
            MATERIAL              103.721     2       51.861    11.153   .003
            METHOD                168.400     4       42.100     9.054   .002

          2-Way Interactions       87.873     8       10.984     2.362   .102
            MATERIAL METHOD        87.873     8       10.984     2.362   .102

          Explained               352.140    14       25.153     5.409   .005

          Residual                 46.500    10        4.650

          Total                   398.640    24       16.610


          25 cases were processed.
          0 cases (.0 pct) were missing.
```

Figure 8.25 Output from **Simple Factorial ANOVA** (with the values of F and their corresponding probabilities highlighted)

From this **Output** it can be seen that there is a significant main effect for the factor material ($P = 0.003$, highlighted in Figure 8.25) and for the factor method ($P = 0.002$). These results should be examined in conjunction with the **Outputs** showing the summary means and standard deviations (Figures 8.20 and 8.22), which help explain the findings. The interaction between the two factors is not significant ($P = 0.102$, highlighted in Figure 8.25).

Representing interactions graphically

To represent interactions graphically, make the selection shown in Figure 8.26.

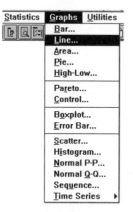

Figure 8.26 Selecting line graphs from the **Graphs** menu

In the next box, select **Multiple** for a graph with multiple lines, as shown in Figure 8.27.

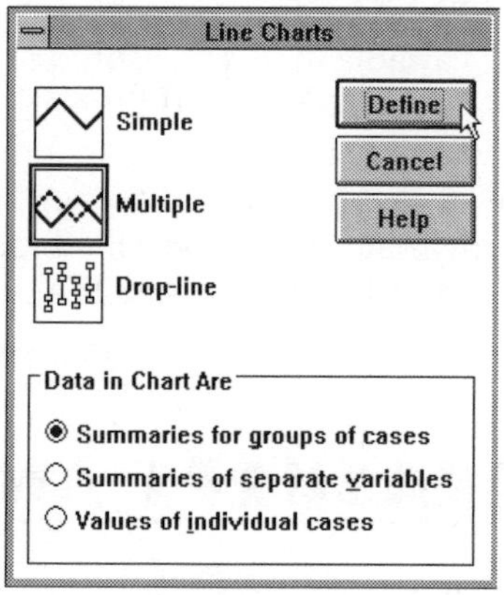

Figure 8.27 Selecting multiple lines in the **Line Charts** box

Click the **Define** button and complete the next box as shown in Figure 8.28. Note that the cell means of the dependent variable, plasticity, will be represented by the lines, while the material has been made the category axis.

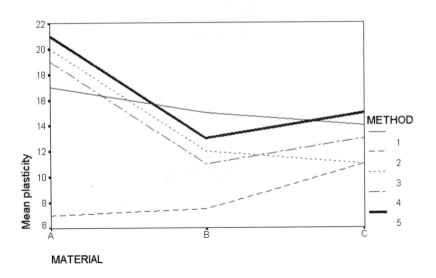

Figure 8.28 Graphical representation of the data of Figure 8.16 (mean plasticity by material and method)

If there were no interaction between the two factors (material and method) the five lines in Figure 8.28 would be parallel. Although this is not the case, they do not strongly deviate from being parallel, in line with the finding that the interaction is not statistically significant.

General factorial ANOVA

A covariate is a concomitant variable that is measured in addition to the dependent variable in ANOVA, and that represents an additional, uncontrolled for, source of variation in the dependent variable. For example, in a psychological study of visual perception, age may be a covariate if it has not been controlled for in the experiment. To allow such covariates to be controlled for in an ANOVA that otherwise fulfills the criteria for a simple factorial ANOVA, it is useful to run a general factorial ANOVA instead.

REPEATED MEASURES ANOVA

The repeated measures ANOVA is used to test hypotheses about the means of a dependent variable when the same dependent variable is measured on more than one occasion for each subject.

Definitions

Between-subjects variables are factors that subdivide the sample into discrete subgroups. Each subject can have only one value for a between-subjects factor.

Within-subjects (repeated measures) variables are factors whose levels are all measured on the same subject.

Mixed (split-plot) design experiments have a mixture of the above two types of variables. Care must be taken in the design of such experiments to reduce carry-over and order effects, for example by counterbalancing.

PARAMETRIC TESTS

Parametric tests are generalizations of the paired samples t-test (see Chapter 6), testing the sources of variation among a group of related dependent variables that represent different measurements of the same attribute.

Mauchly sphericity test and Greenhouse–Geisser epsilon

The criteria that need to be fulfilled to use a repeated measures ANOVA include those listed under Assumptions in the above section on one-way ANOVA, with the obvious exception that repeated measures are now allowed.

In addition, there is also an assumption that the covariance matrix of the transformed variables has a constant variance on the diagonal and zeros off the diagonal. This is tested for using the Mauchly sphericity test. If this test is significant ($P < 0.05$) then the probabilities associated with the values of F from the repeated measures ANOVA should be corrected. This is carried out by multiplying the degrees of freedom (of both the numerator and denominator of the test) by the value of Greenhouse–Geisser epsilon. SPSS gives the value of the latter, and also offers the choice of automatically carrying out this calculation for within-subjects tests, as illustrated in the example that follows.

Procedure

Figure 8.29 shows part of a data file from a study of human visual motion perception, in which sex represents the gender of the subjects, and mot_1 to mot_4 inclusive represent the scores on four successive repeated tests of visual motion. We shall use a repeated measures ANOVA to test whether the visual motion scores vary significantly across the four repeated measures and across gender, and whether there is an interaction between these.

	sex	mot_1	mot_2	mot_3	mot_4
1	Male	15.75	14.03	9.64	12.14
2	Male	15.75	13.24	9.64	11.88
3	Male	6.43	22.27	14.44	7.22
4	Male	18.73	19.28	12.14	26.49
5	Male	5.26	9.92	13.63	8.84
6	Male	19.28	28.88	22.93	16.21
7	Male	10.07	5.25	7.22	7.22
8	Female	25.60	15.75	28.83	17.95

Figure 8.29 Part of a data file from a study of visual motion perception

Repeated measures ANOVA is selected as shown in Figure 8.30.

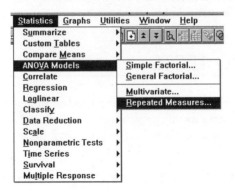

Figure 8.30 Selecting repeated measures ANOVA

This opens the **Repeated Measures Define Factor(s)** box shown in Figure 8.31.

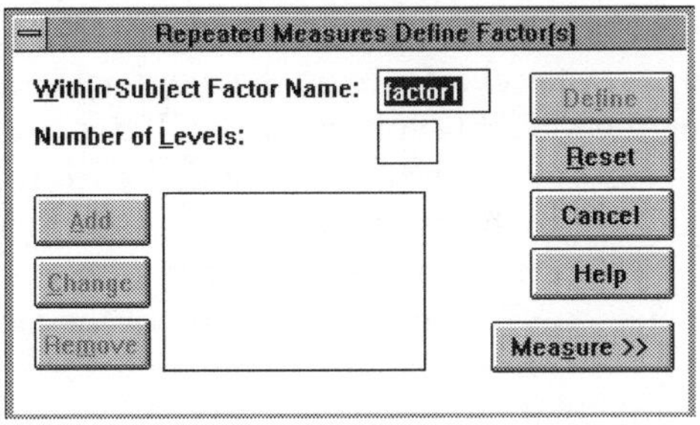

Figure 8.31 The **Repeated Measures Define Factor(s)** box

This is completed as shown in Figure 8.32, from which it can be seen that the name of the within-subject factor (that is, the dependent variable) has been given as 'motion', and four levels (mot_1 to mot_4) have been entered.

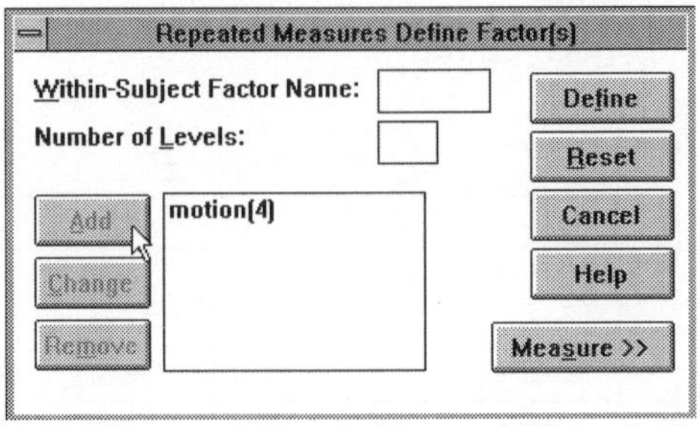

Figure 8.32 Completed **Repeated Measures Define Factor(s)** box

Clicking the **Define** button leads to the **Repeated Measures ANOVA** box, as shown in Figure 8.33.

This box allows you to specify the tests in which you are interested. The Within-Subjects Variables list contains a list of all combinations of factor levels and measures that were defined in the Define Factors box. Each combination is preceded by a blank with a question mark in it. The completed Repeated Measures ANOVA box is shown in Figure 8.34, with mot_1 to mot_4 as the four levels of the within-subject factor (dependent variable) motion, and sex as a between-subjects factor.

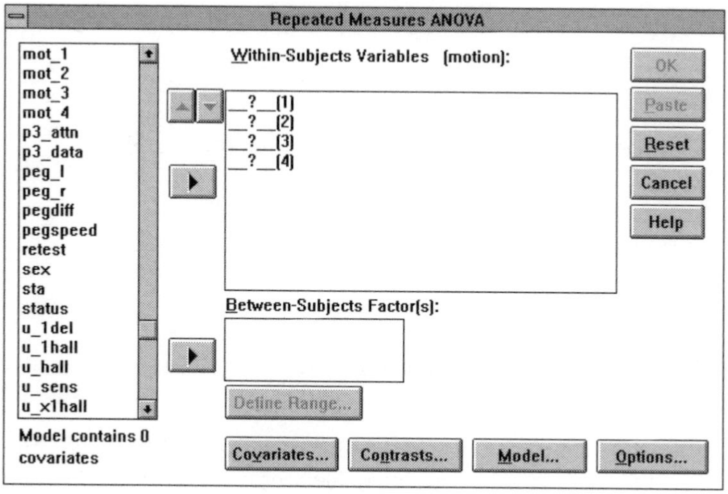

Figure 8.33 The Repeated Measures ANOVA box

Click the Model... button and in the resulting box deselect Multivariate tests in the Within-Subjects Tests group, as shown in Figure 8.35.

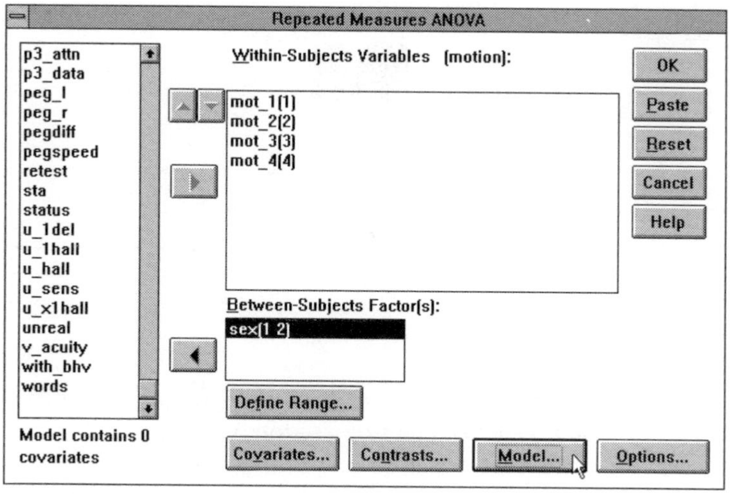

Figure 8.34 Completed Repeated Measures ANOVA box

Clicking Continue returns you to the Repeated Measures ANOVA box. Click OK to obtain the Output. Figure 8.36 shows part of the Output containing the results of the

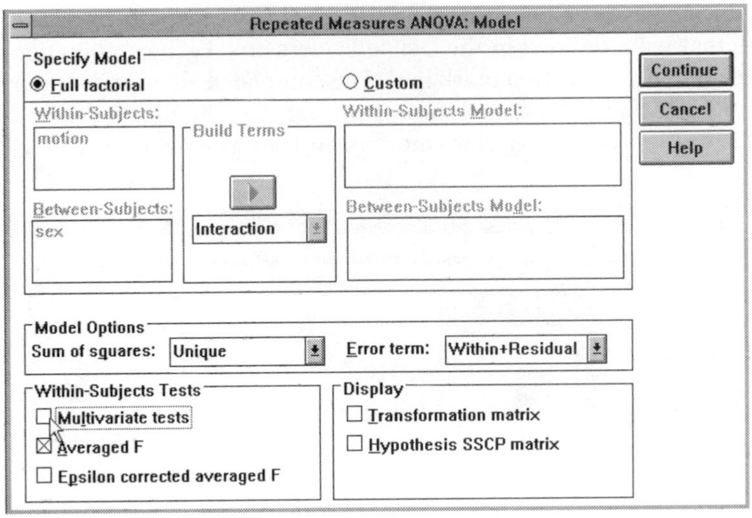

Figure 8.35 The Repeated Measures ANOVA: Model box with Multivariate tests deselected

Mauchly sphericity test, which is seen to be significant ($P = 0.028$, highlighted in Figure 8.36) and the value of Greenhouse–Geisser epsilon (0.74116, highlighted).

Figure 8.36 Output showing the results of the Mauchly sphericity test (significance highlighted) and the value of Greenhouse–Geisser epsilon (highlighted)

The last part of the Output, shown in Figure 8.37, contains the results of the ANOVA, based on uncorrected degrees of freedom (highlighted).

```
_ _ _ _ _ _ _ _ _ _ _ _ _ _ _ _ _ _ _ _ _ _ _ _ _ _ _ _ _ _ _ _ _ _ _ _

|

* * * * * A n a l y s i s   o f   V a r i a n c e -- design   1 * * * * * *

Tests involving 'MOTION' Within-Subject Effect.

AVERAGED Tests of Significance for MOT  using UNIQUE sums of squares
Source of Variation          SS       DF        MS         F  Sig of F

WITHIN+RESIDUAL          1105.57       60     18.43
MOTION                     56.19        3     18.73      1.02     .392
SEX BY MOTION              61.55        3     20.52      1.11     .351

_ _ _ _ _ _ _ _ _ _ _ _ _ _ _ _ _ _ _ _ _ _ _ _ _ _ _ _ _ _ _ _ _ _ _ _
```

Figure 8.37 Output showing the results of the ANOVA (degrees of freedom highlighted)

Since the Mauchly sphericity test is significant, the degrees of freedom highlighted in Figure 8.37 need to be multiplied by the value of Greenhouse-Geisser epsilon (0.74116) and new corresponding significance values of F calculated. (If the Mauchly sphericity test were not significant the results in Figure 8.37 could be taken as the final ones for this ANOVA.) This is readily accomplished by returning to the Repeated Measures ANOVA: Model box and selecting Epsilon corrected averaged F in the Within-Subjects Tests group, as shown in Figure 8.38.

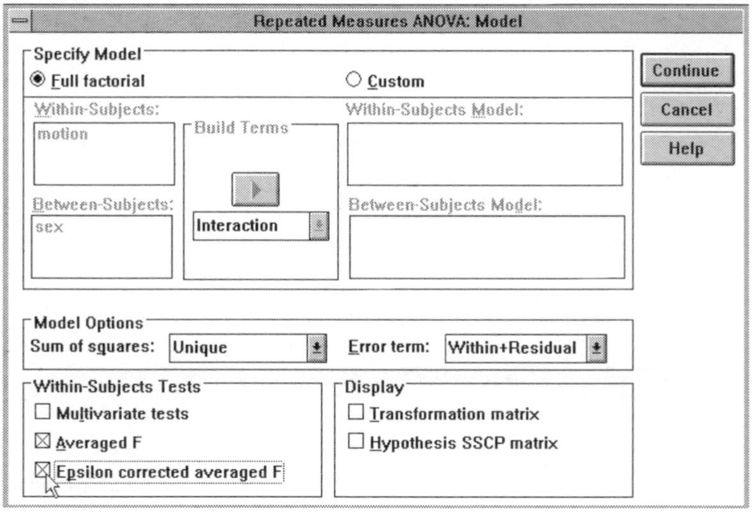

Figure 8.38 The Repeated Measures ANOVA: Model box with Epsilon corrected averaged F selected

Rerunning the ANOVA now results in the Output shown in Figure 8.39.

```
* * * * * A n a l y s i s   o f   V a r i a n c e -- design  1 * * * * * *

Tests involving 'MOTION' Within-Subject Effect.

AVERAGED Tests of Significance for MOT_ using UNIQUE sums of squares
Source of Variation          SS        DF        MS         F  Sig of F

WITHIN+RESIDUAL           1105.57       60      18.43
   (Greenhouse-Geisser)             44.47
   (Huynh-Feldt)                    52.78
   (Lower bound)                    20.00
MOTION                      56.19        3      18.73      1.02     .392
   (Greenhouse-Geisser)              2.22                  1.02     .377
   (Huynh-Feldt)                     2.64                  1.02     .386
   (Lower bound)                     1.00                  1.02     .325
SEX BY MOTION               61.55        3      20.52      1.11     .351
   (Greenhouse-Geisser)              2.22                  1.11     .342
   (Huynh-Feldt)                     2.64                  1.11     .347
   (Lower bound)                     1.00                  1.11     .304
```

Figure 8.39 Output showing the results of the ANOVA (**Epsilon corrected averaged F results for the within-subjects factor motion** highlighted)

In Figure 8.39 the Epsilon corrected averaged F results for the within-subjects factor motion are highlighted. It can be seen that the corresponding significance value is $P = 0.377$. Similarly, Figure 8.40 shows the same Output, but with the Epsilon corrected averaged F results for the sex by motion interaction highlighted.

```
|
* * * * * * A n a l y s i s   o f   V a r i a n c e -- design  1 * * * * * *

Tests involving 'MOTION' Within-Subject Effect.

AVERAGED Tests of Significance for MOT_ using UNIQUE sums of squares
Source of Variation          SS        DF        MS         F  Sig of F

WITHIN+RESIDUAL           1105.57       60      18.43
   (Greenhouse-Geisser)             44.47
   (Huynh-Feldt)                    52.78
   (Lower bound)                    20.00
MOTION                      56.19        3      18.73      1.02     .392
   (Greenhouse-Geisser)              2.22                  1.02     .377
   (Huynh-Feldt)                     2.64                  1.02     .386
   (Lower bound)                     1.00                  1.02     .325
SEX BY MOTION               61.55        3      20.52      1.11     .351
   (Greenhouse-Geisser)              2.22                  1.11     .342
   (Huynh-Feldt)                     2.64                  1.11     .347
   (Lower bound)                     1.00                  1.11     .304
```

Figure 8.40 Output showing the results of the ANOVA (**Epsilon corrected averaged F results for the sex by motion interaction** highlighted)

It can be seen that the corresponding significance value is $P = 0.342$. The results for the between-subjects factor sex are highlighted in the Tests of Between-Subjects Effects given earlier in the Output, and shown in Figure 8.41.

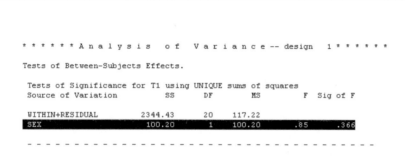

```
* * * * * A n a l y s i s   o f   V a r i a n c e -- design  1 * * * * * *

Tests of Between-Subjects Effects.

  Tests of Significance for T1 using UNIQUE sums of squares
  Source of Variation          SS       DF        MS        F   Sig of F

  WITHIN+RESIDUAL          2344.43       20    117.22
  SEX                      100.20         1    100.20      .85     .366
```

Figure 8.41 Output showing the results of the ANOVA (the results for the **between-subjects factor sex** highlighted)

It can be seen that the corresponding significance value is $P = 0.366$.

Since none of the last three significance values is less than 0.05, there is no evidence that the motion or sex factors have significant main effects. The interaction between motion and sex is also not significant.

NON-PARAMETRIC TESTS

Friedman test

This nonparametric test ranks each variable from 1 to k, where k is the number of variables. The mean rank is then calculated for each variable over all the cases. A test statistic is calculated which has an approximately chi-square distribution and which is used to test the null hypothesis that the k related variables come from the same population. This test is therefore suitable for data that are measured on at least an ordinal scale. The following example gives its use for carrying out an ANOVA with ordinal data.

Seven patients undergo a magnetic resonance imaging (MRI) scan of their brains twice each, the first at the onset of a certain brain disorder, and the second six months later. The images are coregistered, with the baseline scans being subtracted from the second scans for each patient. Three different raters are asked independently to rank the resulting MRI results (mri_1 to mri_7) from 1 (highest amount of change) to 7 (least amount of change). The results are shown in Figure 8.42.

	mri_1	mri_2	mri_3	mri_4	mri_5	mri_6	mri_7
1	1	3	5	2	7	6	4
2	3	2	7	4	6	1	5
3	1	5	3	7	4	6	2

Figure 8.42 Data file showing the ranking of MRI results (mri_1 to mri_7) from 1 (highest amount of change) to 7 (least amount of change) by three independent raters

Nonparametric Tests: K Related Samples is selected as shown in Figure 8.43.

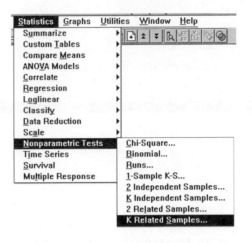

Figure 8.43 Selecting **Nonparametric Tests: K Related Samples**

The resulting box is completed as shown in Figure 8.44.

Tests for Several Related Samples

Test Variables:
mri_1
mri_2
mri_3
mri_4
mri_5
mri_6
mri_7

OK
Paste
Reset
Cancel
Help

Test Type
☒ Friedman   ☐ Kendall's W   ☐ Cochran's Q   Statistics...

Figure 8.44 The **Tests for Several Related Samples** box with the Friedman test selected

Click on **OK** to obtain the **Output** shown in Figure 8.45.

```
- - - - - Friedman Two-Way Anova


Mean Rank    Variable

    1.67     MRI_1
    3.33     MRI_2
    5.00     MRI_3
    4.33     MRI_4
    5.67     MRI_5
    4.33     MRI_6
    3.67     MRI_7

    Cases        Chi-Square        D.F.    Significance
      3           6.4286            6        3.77E-01
```

Figure 8.45 Output showing the results of the Friedman ANOVA (significance highlighted)

The probability corresponding to the test statistic has been highlighted (P = 3.77E–01 = 3.77×10^{-1} = 0.377) and so the rankings of the seven MRI results are not significantly different.

Kendall's W test

Kendall's W test is a nonparametric test which ranks each variable from 1 to k, where k is the number of variables. The mean rank is then calculated for each variable over all the cases. Kendall's W and the corresponding chi-square statistic are then calculated, with ties corrected for. The latter is used to test the null hypothesis that the k related variables come from the same population. This test is therefore suitable for data that are measured on at least an ordinal scale.

W tests for agreement of the rankings by the judges or raters and ranges from 0 (no agreement) to 1 (complete agreement). Each case is assumed to be a judge or rater. Thus Kendall's W test is useful for testing inter-rater reliability.

To determine the value of Kendall's W for the three raters in the previous example (Figure 8.42), complete the Tests for Several Related Samples box in the way shown in Figure 8.46.

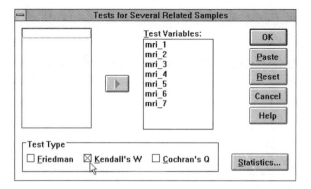

Figure 8.46 The Tests for Several Related Samples box with Kendall's W test selected

Cochran's Q test

When OK is clicked, the resulting Output is as shown in Figure 8.47.

```
- - - - - Kendall Coefficient of Concordance


  Mean Rank    Variable

      1.67     MRI_1
      3.33     MRI_2
      5.00     MRI_3
      4.33     MRI_4
      5.67     MRI_5
      4.33     MRI_6
      3.67     MRI_7


    Cases          W          Chi-Square     D.F.   Significance
        3       3.571E-01        6.4286         6      3.77E-01
```

Figure 8.47 Output showing the results of Kendall's W test (W highlighted)

The mean rank for each variable is the same as in Figure 8.45, as is the value of chi-square. The value of Kendall's W (for the three raters) is highlighted and is $3.571E{-}01 = 3.571 \times 10^{-1} = 0.3571$.

This tests the null hypothesis that the proportion of cases in a particular category is the same for several dichotomous variables. It is suitable for use when there are related samples measured on dichotomous (binary) nominal scales.

Suppose that in the previous example the three raters were asked simply to rate whether they considered significant change had occurred in the MRI results (rated as 1) or not (rated as 0). The corresponding data file is shown in Figure 8.48.

	mri_1	mri_2	mri_3	mri_4	mri_5	mri_6	mri_7
1	1	1	0	1	0	0	0
2	1	1	0	1	0	1	0
3	1	0	1	0	0	0	1

Figure 8.48 Data file showing the dichotomous ratings of MRI results (mri_1 to mri_7) as either 0 (no significant change) or 1 (significant change) by three independent raters

Complete the Tests for Several Related Samples box in the way shown in Figure 8.49.

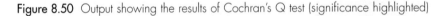

Figure 8.49 The Tests for Several Related Samples box with Cochran's Q test selected

When **OK** is clicked, the resulting Output is as shown in Figure 8.50.

```
- - - - - Cochran Q Test


Cases

= 1   = 0    Variable

   3    0    MRI_1
   2    1    MRI_2
   1    2    MRI_3
   2    1    MRI_4
   0    3    MRI_5
   1    2    MRI_6
   1    2    MRI_7

        Cases        Cochran Q        D.F.   Significance
          3           6.6667            6          .3528
```

Figure 8.50 Output showing the results of Cochran's Q test (significance highlighted)

The probability corresponding to the test statistic has been highlighted ($P = 0.3528$) and so the rankings of the seven MRI results are not significantly different.

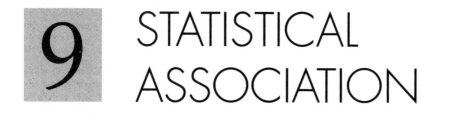

9 STATISTICAL ASSOCIATION

In this chapter we are concerned with bivariate data, that is, sets of data involving observations of two variables.

PARAMETRIC TEST

For interval or ratio data that satisfy the normality assumption (see Chapter 4), the Pearson product moment correlation coefficient, often referred to simply as the correlation coefficient, can be used. If the normality assumption is violated, or the data are not interval or ratio, then a nonparametric test should be considered (described later in this chapter).

Graphical representation

Bivariate data measured on an interval or ratio scale can be represented in the form of scatter diagrams as in Figure 9.1, in which the line of best fit (the linear regression line; see Chapter 10) has been superimposed upon the data.

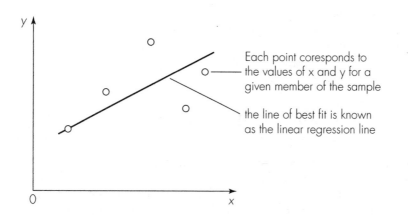

Based on Puri, BK (1996) *Statistics for the Health Sciences*, with permission from WB Saunders, London

Finding a statistical association between two variables does not necessary imply that this association is linear. Graphically, this can be represented by the fact that the line of best fit may not be a straight line. In Figure 9.2, for example, the line of best fit is cubic.

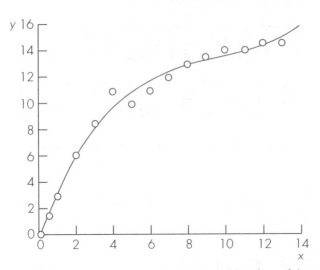

Figure 9.2 A scatter diagram of bivariate data with a cubic line of best fit superimposed. Reproduced from Puri, BK (1996) Statistics for the Health Sciences, with permission from Churchill Livingstone, Edinburgh

Pearson product moment correlation coefficient

The Pearson product moment correlation coefficient measures the strength of the linear relationship for bivariate data for the two variables. If the two random variables are positively correlated, they tend to increase or decrease together. If they are negatively correlated, one tends to increase as the other decreases.

The value of the Pearson correlation coefficient varies between –1 and 1 inclusive, and does not have any units. Figure 9.3 shows typical scatter diagrams for the range of possible values of the Pearson correlation coefficient, which is denoted by r when obtained from a sample. (The corresponding population correlation coefficient is denoted by ρ.) The range of values is as follows:

- $r = 1$: perfect positive correlation
- $0 < r < 1$: positive though not perfect correlation
- $r = 0$: no correlation
- $-1 < r < 0$: negative though not perfect correlation
- $= -1$: perfect negative correlation

Scatter plot of the bivariate data

It is useful to plot the data in the form of a scatter diagram for the following reasons:

- it provides a useful check on the range in which the correlation coefficient should lie (see Figure 9.3)
- it indicates the presence of any outliers; if these are present their data values should be carefully rechecked in the data file and if correct there should be checked in the raw data (the correlation coefficient procedure may have to be rerun without the outlier(s))
- it may indicate the shape of the line of best fit, which may not be a straight line but, for example, curved as in Figure 9.2
- if the line of best fit is not linear, an indication may be given of the type of data transformation that may make it linear.

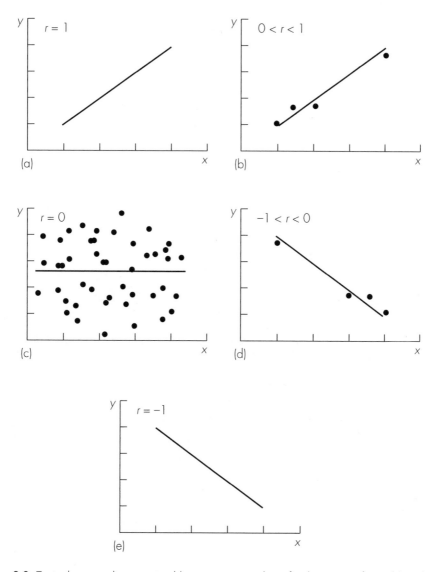

Figure 9.3 Typical scatter diagrams and linear regression lines for the range of possible values of the Pearson product moment correlation coefficient, *r*. (a) *r* = 1; (b) 0 < *r* < 1; (c) *r* = 0; (d) −1 < *r* < 0; (e) *r* = −1. Based on Puri BK (1996) *Statistics for the Health Sciences*, with permission from WB Saunders, London

The way in which scatterplots are produced for bivariate data has been explained in Chapter 6 (Figures 6.12–6.15).

Procedure

Figure 9.4 shows the data file of the cerebrospinal fluid levels of 5-HIAA (5-hydroxy-indoleacetic acid) and cortisol in 14 untreated patients suffering from depression. We wish to determine the value of the Pearson product moment correlation coefficient for these two substances in this group of patients.

	hiaa	cortisol
1	100	38
2	52	25
3	50	27
4	48	18
5	124	29
6	167	39
7	147	26
8	112	35
9	102	31
10	148	33
11	70	26
12	58	28
13	97	24
14	120	31

Figure 9.4 Data file of the cerebrospinal fluid levels of 5-HIAA and cortisol in 14 untreated depressed patients (both measured in units of nmol 1^{-1} = nM)

The first thing to do is to produce a scatterplot of this set of bivariate data. This is shown in Figure 9.5.

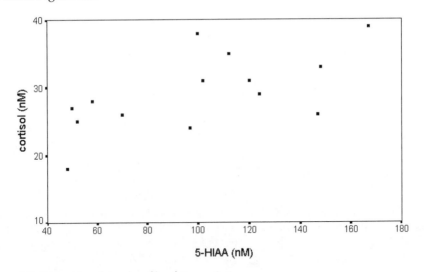

Figure 9.5 Scatterplot of the data file of Figure 9.4

From this scatterplot we can see that the correlation coefficient will lie between 0 and 1 (both exclusive), that there are no obvious outliers, and that it is reasonable to have a line of best fit that is linear.

Check that the normality assumption holds for both variables (see Chapter 4). If it does not, then consider using a nonparametric test (such as the Spearman rank correlation or Kendall's tau-b) instead; these are described later in this chapter.

To determine the actual value of the correlation coefficient, make the selection shown in Figure 9.6.

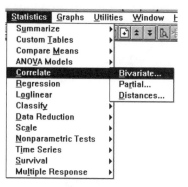

Figure 9.6 Selecting bivariate correlations

The resulting **Bivariate Correlations** box is completed as shown in Figure 9.7.

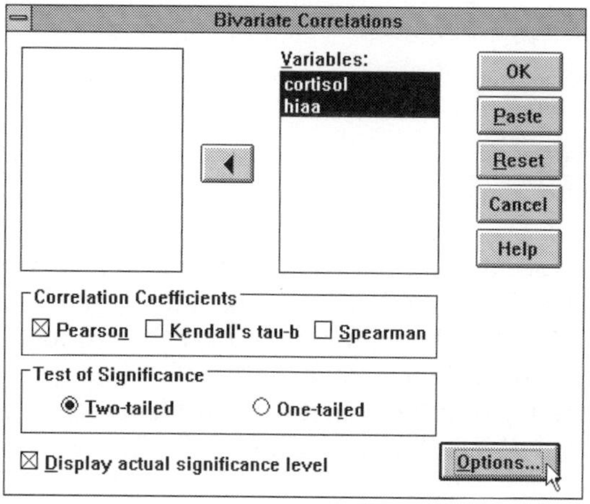

Figure 9.7 The **Bivariate Correlations** box (selecting the **Pearson correlation coefficient**)

If you would like the values of the means and standard deviations of the two variables to be calculated as well, click the Options... button and complete the next box, as shown in Figure 9.8.

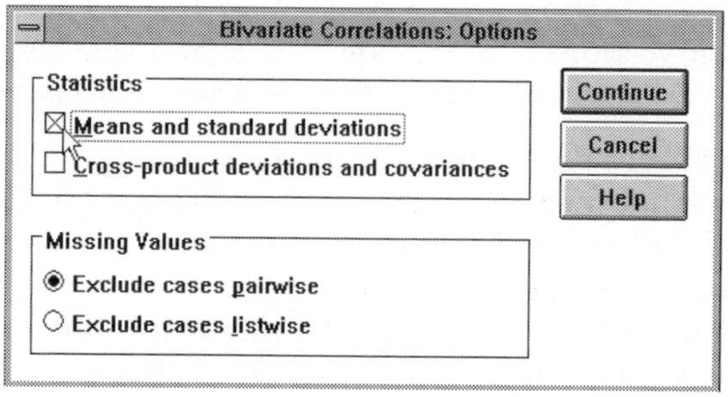

Figure 9.8 The **Bivariate Correlations: Options** box

Click on **Continue** to return to the previous box, and then on **OK** to obtain the **Output**, shown in Figure 9.9.

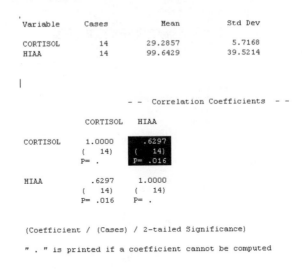

```
 Variable      Cases          Mean          Std Dev

 CORTISOL       14          29.2857          5.7168
 HIAA           14          99.6429         39.5214


 |

                        - -  Correlation Coefficients  - -

                     CORTISOL   HIAA

 CORTISOL            1.0000      .6297
                     (    14)    (    14)
                     P= .        P= .016


 HIAA                 .6297     1.0000
                     (    14)   (    14)
                     P= .016    P= .


 (Coefficient / (Cases) / 2-tailed Significance)

 " . " is printed if a coefficient cannot be computed
```

Figure 9.9 Output showing means, standard deviations and Pearson product moment correlation coefficient (highlighted) for the data file of Figure 9.4

From this **Output** we can see that for the 5-HIAA the mean level is 99.6429 nM with a standard deviation of 39.5214 nM. For the cortisol the mean level is 29.2857 nM, standard deviation 5.7168 nM. The value of the Pearson product moment correlation coefficient is 0.6297 (highlighted in Figure 9.9), based on 14 pairs of cases (highlighted – it appears in parentheses in the **Output**). This correlation coefficient is significant at the 5% level ($P = 0.016$; highlighted).

NONPARAMETRIC TESTS

Ordinal data

For bivariate data that are measured on at least an ordinal scale (that is, ordinal, interval or ratio), SPSS offers the following two nonparametric tests:

● Spearman's rank correlation, which uses differences between pairs of ranks to give a nonparametric version of the Pearson product moment correlation coefficient.
● Kendall's tau-b, which is similar to Spearman's rank correlation.

The values of both Spearman's rank correlation and Kendall's tau-b lie in the same range as the Pearson product moment correlation coefficient (between –1 and 1, both inclusive), and their values have similar meanings (a value of 1 implies perfect positive correlation, and so on).

As when determining the Pearson product moment correlation coefficient, it is useful to produce a scatterplot, for the reasons given above.

To illustrate the use of these nonparametric tests, let us suppose the data in Figure 9.4 violated the normality assumption so that we could not use the Pearson correlation coefficient. (As we have already produced a scatterplot (Figure 9.5) and considered its implications, we shall not do so again now.)

Complete the Bivariate Correlations box (selected as in Figure 9.6) as shown in Figure 9.10.

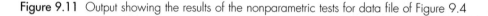

```
┌─────────────────────────────────────────────────────┐
│ ▄                 Bivariate Correlations          ▲  │
│ ╔══════════════╗   Variables:         ┌──────────┐   │
│ ║              ║   cortisol           │   OK   ▛ │   │
│ ║              ║   hiaa               └──────────┘   │
│ ║              ║                      ┌──────────┐   │
│ ║              ║                      │  Paste   │   │
│ ║              ║   ┌───┐              └──────────┘   │
│ ║              ║   │ ▶ │              ┌──────────┐   │
│ ║              ║   └───┘              │  Reset   │   │
│ ║              ║                      └──────────┘   │
│ ║              ║                      ┌──────────┐   │
│ ║              ║                      │ Cancel   │   │
│ ╚══════════════╝                      └──────────┘   │
│                                       ┌──────────┐   │
│                                       │  Help    │   │
│  ┌Correlation Coefficients────────────┴──────────┴─┐ │
│  │ ☐ Pearson  ☒ Kendall's tau-b  ☒ Spearman       │ │
│  └──────────────────────────────────────────────────┘ │
│  ┌Test of Significance──────────────────────────────┐ │
│  │ ◉ Two-tailed        ○ One-tailed                 │ │
│  └──────────────────────────────────────────────────┘ │
│  ☒ Display actual significance level    ┌─────────┐  │
│                                          │Options..│  │
│                                          └─────────┘  │
└─────────────────────────────────────────────────────┘
```

Figure 9.10 The **Bivariate Correlations** box (selecting the nonparametric tests)

Click **OK** to obtain the **Output** shown in Figure 9.11.

```
- - - - K E N D A L L   C O R R E L A T I O N   C O E F F I C I E N T S   - - -


HIAA              .4556
               N(   14)
               Sig .024


               CORTISOL

(Coefficient / (Cases) / 2-tailed Significance)

" . " is printed if a coefficient cannot be computed




- - - S P E A R M A N   C O R R E L A T I O N   C O E F F I C I E N T S   - - -


HIAA              .6520
               N(   14)
               Sig .012


               CORTISOL

(Coefficient / (Cases) / 2-tailed Significance)

" . " is printed if a coefficient cannot be computed
```

Figure 9.11 Output showing the results of the nonparametric tests for data file of Figure 9.4

From this **Output** it can be seen that the value of Kendall's tau-b is 0.4556 (based on 14 pairs of cases) and that this value is significant (P = 0.024). The value of Spearman's rank correlation is 0.6520, which is also significant (P = 0.012).

Nominal data

Unless the nominal data have a meaningful order (categorical data), no meaning can be attached to a direction of association; rather, the strength of association between two nominal variables is all that can be measured.

SPSS offers the following three measures of association based on the chi-square statistic:

- The phi coefficient. Phi is calculated by dividing the value of chi-square by the sample size and then taking the square root of the result. For 2×2 contingency tables SPSS gives phi the same sign as the Pearson correlation coefficient, and its range is from –1 to 1. For tables with more than two rows and/or more than two columns, however, phi can, unfortunately, have a value greater than 1.
- Cramér's V. V is calculated by dividing the value of chi-square by both the sample size and the smaller of the number of rows and columns, and then taking the square root of the result. V always lies between 0 and 1 (inclusive) and can attain a value of 1 for tables of any dimension (unlike the contingency coefficient described next).
- Contingency coefficient. This is calculated by dividing the value of chi-square by the sum of chi-square and the sample size, and then taking the square root of the result. It always lies between 0 and 1, but it is not generally possible to attain the value 1, even for a contingency table showing a perfect relationship. The maximum value depends on the number of rows and columns in the contingency table.

Let us return to the example shown in Figure 7.3, which shows part of a data file from a study on dyslexia, with dyslexic status (normal control or dyslexic) and handedness group (right consistent, mixed preference or left consistent) highlighted. For these two variables we shall determine the values of the above three measures of association.

Follow the steps shown in Figures 7.4 and 7.5 to obtain the Crosstabs: Statistics box. This should be completed as shown in Figure 9.12.

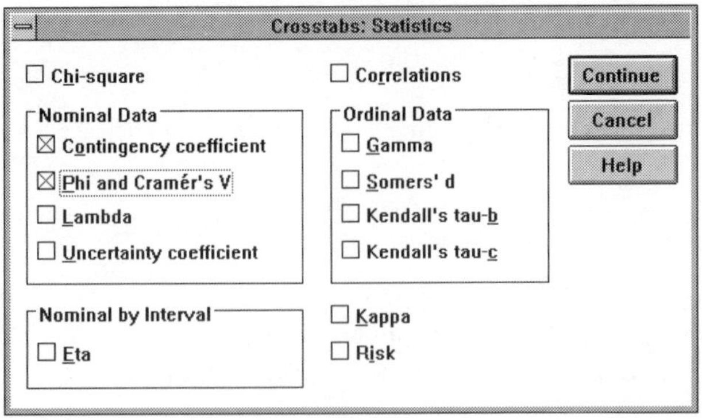

Figure 9.12 The **Crosstabs: Statistics** box with measures of association based on chi-square for nominal data selected

Click **Continue** and then in the next box click **OK** to obtain the **Output** shown in Figure 9.13.

Statistic	Value	ASE1	Val/ASE0	Approximate Significance
Phi	.32581			.00000 *1
Cramer's V	.32581			.00000 *1
Contingency Coefficient	.30978			.00000 *1

```
*1 Pearson chi-square probability

Number of Missing Observations:  0
```

Figure 9.13 Output showing the results of the measures of association based on chi-square for the data file of Figure 7.3

From this **Output** it can be seen that all three measures of association are significant, and have the following values: phi and Cramér's *V* both have the value 0.32581, while the contingency coefficient has the value 0.30978.

10 LINEAR REGRESSION BETWEEN TWO VARIABLES

In this chapter linear regression between two variables is described. If a scatter diagram shows a non-linear relationship between the two variables (see Chapter 9), then it may be possible to use data transformation (see Chapter 5) to convert this into a linear relationship.

STRAIGHT LINE EQUATION

Any straight line can be represented by means of the equation $y = a + bx$, where y is the dependent variable, a is the intercept on the y-axis, b is the gradient of the line, and x is the independent variable. These are shown in Figure 10.1, in which the gradient is positive (and therefore the value of b is positive).

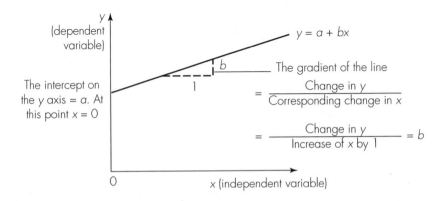

Figure 10.1 The graph of a straight line with positive gradient. Based on Puri, BK (1996) *Statistics for the Health Sciences*, with permission from WB Saunders, London

The gradient of the straight line in Figure 10.2 is negative (and therefore the value of b is negative).

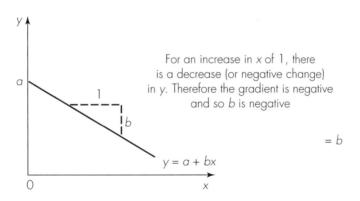

Figure 10.2 The graph of a straight line with negative gradient. Based on Puri, BK (1996) *Statistics for the Health Sciences*, with permission from WB Saunders, London

If the gradient of the linear regression line is zero, that is the line is horizontal (and therefore the value of *b* is zero), there is no linear relationship between the two variables.

LEAST SQUARES METHOD

In order to determine the line of best fit for bivariate data the least squares method is used. This is shown in Figure 10.3.

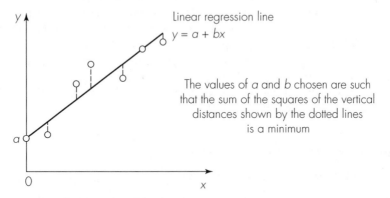

Figure 10.3 The method of least squares to determine the linear regression line. Based on Puri, BK (1996) *Statistics for the Health Sciences*, with permission from WB Saunders, London

ASSUMPTIONS

Assumptions made in linear regression include the following.

- There is no error in the observed values of the independent variable, *x*.
- For any value of *x* there is a normal distribution of values of *y* (see Figure 10.4); these normal distributions for different values of *x* have the same standard deviation.

● The true mean of each y from these normal distributions (for example y_1 and y_2 in Figure 10.4) lies on the linear regression line.

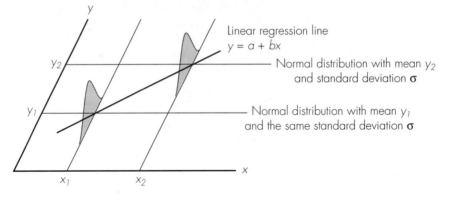

Figure 10.4 Some of the assumptions made in using linear regression. Based on Puri BK and Tyrer P (1992) *Sciences Basic to Psychiatry*, with permission from Churchill Livingstone, Edinburgh

PROCEDURE

As mentioned in the last chapter, it is useful to produce a scatter plot of a set of bivariate data. Amongst other things, this helps to indicate whether or not the shape of the line of best fit is linear, as well as indicating whether there are any outliers (see Chapter 9).

In the previous chapter, Figure 9.4 showed a data file of the cerebrospinal fluid levels of 5-HIAA (5-hydroxyindoleacetic acid) and cortisol in 14 untreated patients suffering from depression. (The Pearson product moment correlation coefficient for these two substances in this group of patients was determined.) We shall determine the equation of the linear regression line for these data, and superimpose this line on the scatterplot of the data (shown in Figure 9.5).

From this scatterplot we can see that there are no obvious outliers and that it is reasonable to have a line of best fit that is linear.

Linear regression equation

Make the selection shown in Figure 10.5.

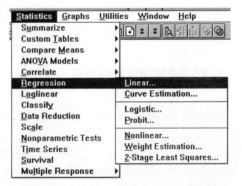

Figure 10.5 Selecting linear regression

Complete the resulting linear regression box, as shown in Figure 10.6.

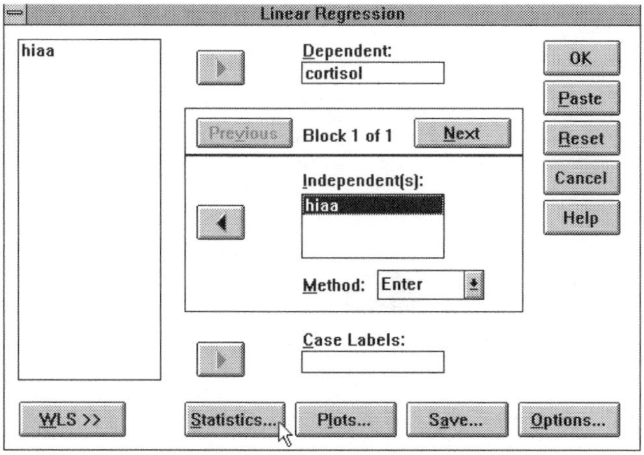

Figure 10.6 The Linear Regression box

Click the Statistics... button and in the next box select any additional statistics you require in addition to or instead of the default selections (Estimates of Regression Coefficients and Model fit). In this case we have additionally selected Confidence Intervals of the Regression Coefficients and Descriptives, as shown in Figure 10.7.

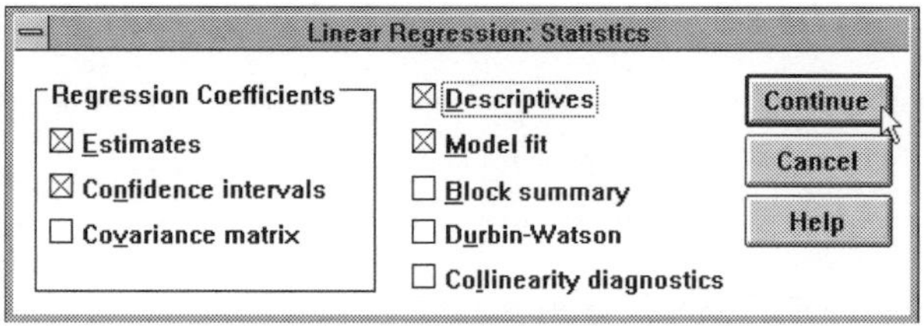

Figure 10.7 The Linear Regression: Statistics box

Click Continue and then in the previous box click OK. The first part of the Output contains the descriptive statistics and the correlation coefficient (with one-tailed significance), as shown in Figure 10.8.

```
              * * * *   M U L T I P L E   R E G R E S S I O N   * * * *

    Listwise Deletion of Missing Data

                    Mean  Std Dev  Label

    CORTISOL    29.286    5.717  cortisol (nM)
    HIAA        99.643   39.521  5-HIAA (nM)

    N of Cases =    14

    Correlation, 1-tailed Sig:

                  CORTISOL        HIAA

    CORTISOL      1.000         .630
                    .            .008

    HIAA           .630        1.000
                   .008           .
```

Figure 10.8 Output from linear regression showing the descriptive statistics and the correlation coefficient (highlighted) with one-tailed significance (highlighted)

It can be seen that the correlation coefficient between the two variables is 0.630, with a one-tailed significance of 0.008, highlighted in Figure 10.8. (Note that in the determination of the correlation coefficient in Chapter 9, the *two*-tailed significance was calculated.) The next part of the Output contains the Multiple R and a linear regression ANOVA, shown in Figure 10.9.

```
              * * * *   M U L T I P L E   R E G R E S S I O N   * * * *

    Equation Number 1    Dependent Variable..   CORTISOL   cortisol (nM)

       Descriptive Statistics are printed on Page    4

    Block Number  1.  Method:  Enter      HIAA

    Variable(s) Entered on Step Number
       1..    HIAA      5-HIAA (nM)

    Multiple R            .62967
    R Square              .39648
    Adjusted R Square     .34619
    Standard Error       4.62249

    Analysis of Variance
                      DF     Sum of Squares     Mean Square
    Regression         1          168.44866      168.44866
    Residual          12          256.40849       21.36737

    F =     7.88345       Signif F =   .0158
```

Figure 10.9 Output from linear regression showing the Multiple R (highlighted) and a linear regression ANOVA

With the analysis of bivariate data, in which there is just one independent variable, the value of Multiple R is the same as that of the Pearson product moment correlation coefficient between the two variables (highlighted in Figure 10.9). The number directly underneath, R Square, is simply the value of the square of the correlation coefficient (r^2). This is also known as the coefficient of determination and is the proportion of the variation in the observed values of y that can be explained by x and therefore by the linear regression line. In this case the proportion is approximately 39.6% (highlighted in Figure 10.9). The linear regression ANOVA tests whether the relationship between the two variables is linear. This is the case if the value of F is significant (which is the case in Figure 10.9, in which in the last line Signif F = 0.0158) *and* if the scatterplot indicates a linear relationship (which Figure 9.5 does).

The final part of the Output gives the variables in the linear regression equation with their confidence intervals and significances (Figure 10.10).

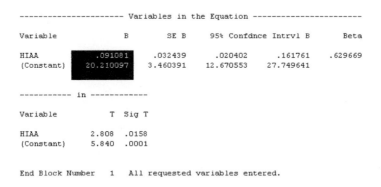

```
---------------------- Variables in the Equation ----------------------

Variable              B        SE B    95% Confdnce Intrvl B      Beta

HIAA                .091081    .032439     .020402     .161761   .629669
(Constant)         20.210097  3.460391   12.670553   27.749641


----------- in ------------

Variable           T   Sig T

HIAA            2.808   .0158
(Constant)      5.840   .0001


End Block Number   1   All requested variables entered.
```

Figure 10.10 Output from linear regression showing the variables in the equation

The highlighted values in Figure 10.10 respectively give the values for b (0.091081) and a (20.210097) in the linear regression equation $y = a + bx$. The next column gives the standard errors for b (0.032439) and a (3.460391). The next two columns give the 95% confidence intervals for b (0.020402 to 0.161761) and a (12.670553 to 27.749641). The last column gives the significance values for b (0.0158) and a (0.0001); both values are clearly significant.

Graph of linear regression line

Earlier in this book we have shown how to produce a scatterplot of bivariate data (see Chapters 6 and 9). In the Chart Carousel containing this scatterplot, press the Edit button shown in Figure 10.11.

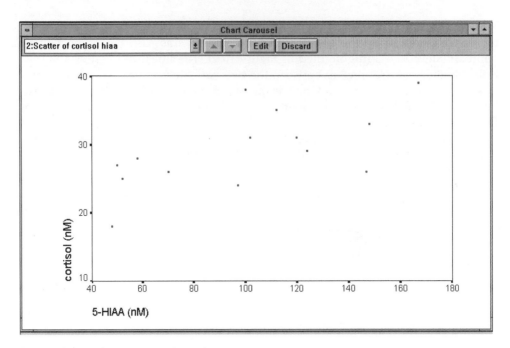

Figure 10.11 Editing a scatterplot in the **Chart Carousel**

The resulting Chart Carousel in Edit mode then appears, as shown in Figure 10.12.

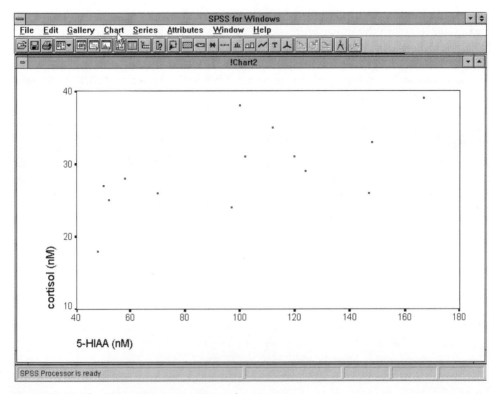

Figure 10.12 The **Chart Carousel** in **Edit** mode

Make the selection shown in Figure 10.13.

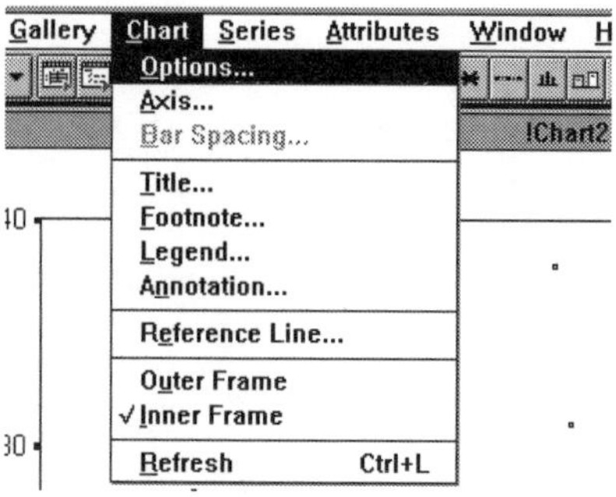

Figure 10.13 Selecting chart options

In the Fit Line group in the resulting box, select Total, as shown in Figure 10.14.

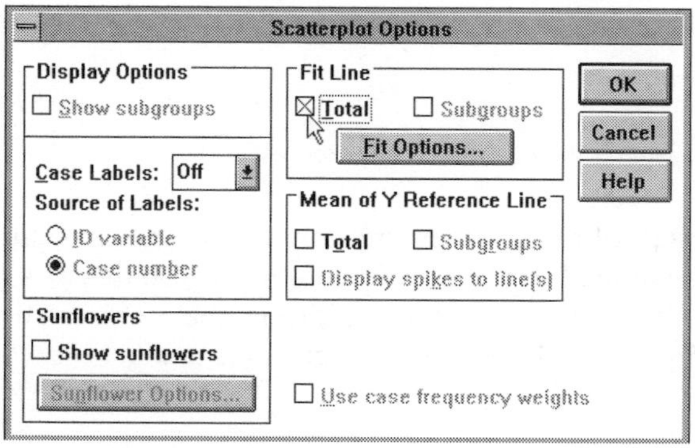

Figure 10.14 The Scatterplot Options box

If you wish to check that linear regression is the default setting, click the Fit Options box to obtain the Scatterplot Options: Fit Line box shown in Figure 10.15.

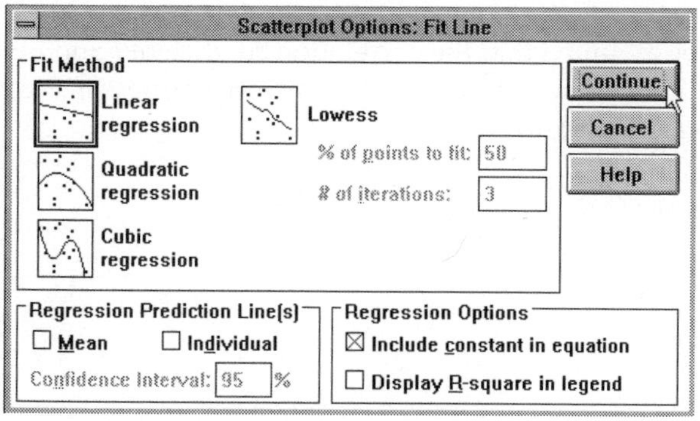

Figure 10.15 The Scatterplot Options: Fit Line box

Click Continue, and then, on returning to the previous box, click OK. This results in a linear regression being superimposed on the scatterplot, as shown in Figure 10.16.

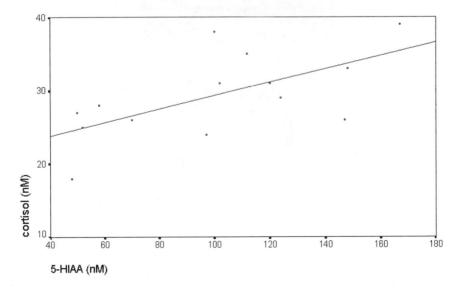

Figure 10.16 Scatterplot with superimposed linear regression line

Note that the intercept of the linear regression line on the left-hand vertical axis is not the same as the value of a (20.210097). This is because this axis is not the true y-axis ($x = 0$) since this chart has started plotting the x-axis at the value 40 nM. However, the chart can readily be edited to give a true y-axis ($x = 0$) if required.

EXTRAPOLATION AND PREDICTION

The linear regression line equation can be used to predict values of y for given values of x. However, this should only be carried out for values of x lying in the range of x used to determine the equation in the first place, and also only if the value of the coefficient of determination r^2 is not close to zero.

Figure 10.17 illustrates why, when a linear correlation is found between two variables, it must not be assumed that the correlation coefficient r and the corresponding linear regression line can be extrapolated to include values of x and y outside the range used in their calculation.

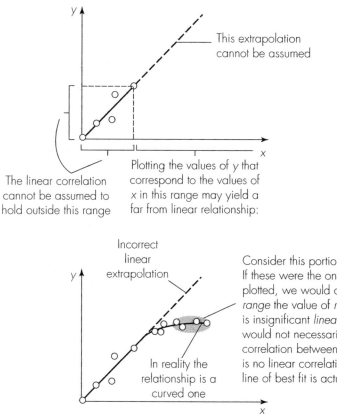

Figure 10.17 Illustration of why extrapolation and prediction may not be valid outside the range used to calculate the correlation coefficient and linear regression equation. Based on Puri, BK (1996) *Statistics for the Health Sciences*, with permission from WB Saunders, London

To plot the 95% confidence interval for the predicted means, return to the **Scatterplot Options: Fit Line** box (Figure 10.15) and make the selection shown in Figure 10.18.

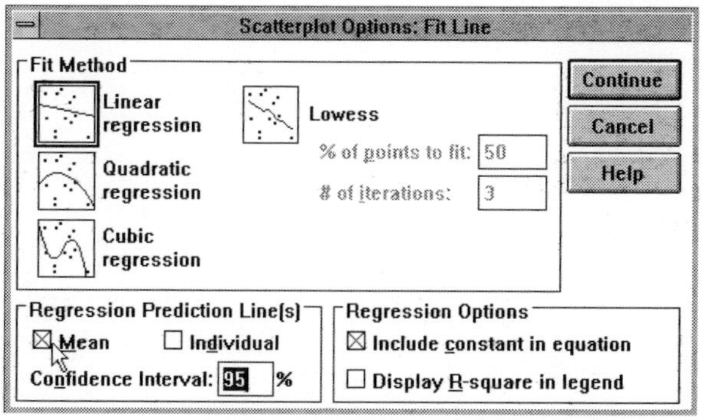

Figure 10.18 The **Scatterplot Options: Fit Line** box – selecting **Mean Regression Predication Line(s)**

The resulting chart, with the linear regression line and the confidence interval for mean prediction, is shown in Figure 10.19.

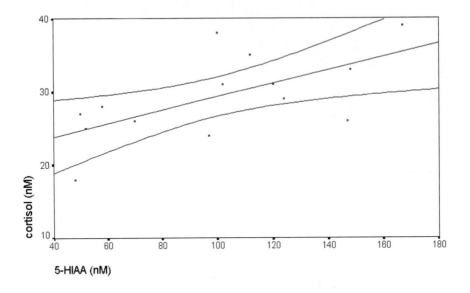

Figure 10.19 Scatterplot with superimposed linear regression line and 95% confidence intervals

APPENDIX

FUNCTIONS AVAILABLE IN THE COMPUTE VARIABLE BOX

ABS(numexpr) *Numeric* Returns the absolute value of numexpr, which must be numeric.

ANY(test,value[,value,...]) *Logical* Returns 1 or true if the value of test matches any of the subsequent values; returns 0 or false otherwise. It requires two or more arguments.

ARSIN(numexpr) *Numeric* Returns the arcsine, in radians, of numexpr, which must evaluate to a numeric value between -1 and +1.

ARTAN(numexpr) *Numeric* Returns the arctangent, in radians, of numexpr, which must be numeric.

CDF.distribution(numexpr, ...) *Numeric* Returns the probability that a random variable with a specified distribution would be less than numexpr.

CDFNORM(zvalue) *Numeric* Returns the probability that a random variable with mean 0 and standard deviation 1 would be less than zvalue, which must be numeric.

CFVAR(numexpr,numexpr[,...]) *Numeric* Returns the coefficient of variation (the standard deviation divided by the mean) of its arguments that have valid values. It requires two or more arguments, which must be numeric.

CONCAT(strexpr,strexpr[,...]) *String* Returns a string that is the concatenation of all its arguments, which must evaluate to strings. It requires two or more arguments.

COS(radians) *Numeric* Returns the cosine of a numeric value measured in radians.

CTIME.DAYS(timevalue) *Numeric* Returns the number of days, including fractional days, in timevalue.

CTIME.HOURS(timevalue) *Numeric* Returns the number of hours, including fractional hours, in timevalue.

CTIME.MINUTES(timevalue) *Numeric* Returns the number of minutes, including fractional minutes, in timevalue.

CTIME.SECONDS(timevalue) *Numeric* Returns the number of seconds, including fractional seconds, in timevalue.

DATE.DMY(day,month,year) *Numeric in SPSS date format* Returns a date value corresponding to the indicated day, month, and year. To display this value correctly, assign it a DATE format. The arguments must be integers, with day between 1 and 31, month between 1 and 13, and year a four-digit integer greater than 1582 or a two-digit integer with an assumed prefix of 19.

DATE.MDY(month,day,year) *Numeric in SPSS date format* Returns a date value corresponding to the indicated month, day, and year. To display this value correctly, assign it a DATE format. Arguments are as in the preceding function.

DATE.MOYR(month,year) *Numeric in SPSS date format* Returns a date value corresponding to the indicated month and year. To display this value correctly, assign it a DATE format. The arguments must be integers, with month between 1 and 13, and year a four-digit integer greater than 1582 or a two-digit integer with an assumed prefix of 19.

DATE.QYR(quarter,year) *Numeric in SPSS date format* Returns a date value corresponding to the indicated quarter and year. To display this value correctly, assign it a DATE format. The arguments must be integers, with quarter between 1 and 4, and year a 4-digit integer greater than 1582 or a 2-digit integer with an assumed prefix of 19.

DATE.WKYR(weeknum,year) *Numeric in SPSS date format* Returns a date value corresponding to the indicated weeknum and year. To display this value correctly, assign it a DATE format. The arguments must be integers, with weeknum between 1 and 52, and year a four-digit integer greater than 1582 or a two-digit integer with an assumed prefix of 19.

DATE.YRDAY(year,daynum) *Numeric in SPSS date format* Returns a date value corresponding to the indicated year and daynum. To display this value correctly, assign it a DATE format. The arguments must be integers, with daynum between 1 and 366, and year a four-digit integer greater than 1582 or a two-digit integer with an assumed prefix of 19.

EXP(numexpr) *Numeric* Returns e raised to the power numexpr, where numexpr is numeric.

IDF.distribution(prob, ...) *Numeric* Returns the value in a specified distribution with a cumulative probability equal to prob.

INDEX(haystack,needle) *Numeric* Returns an integer that indicates the starting position of the first occurrence of the string needle in the string haystack. Returns 0 if needle does not occur within haystack.

INDEX(haystack,needle,divisor) *Numeric* See the preceding function. The optional third argument divisor is the number of characters used to divide needle into separate strings to be sought. It must be an integer that divides evenly into the length of needle.

LAG(variable) *Numeric or string* Returns the value of variable for the previous case in the data file. Returns system-missing (numeric variables) or blank (string variables) for the first case.

LAG(variable,ncases) *Numeric or string* Returns the value of variable for the case that is ncases earlier in the file. Returns system-missing (numeric variables) or blank (string variables) for the first ncases cases.

LENGTH(strexpr) *Numeric* Returns the length of strexpr, which must be a string expression. This is the defined length, including trailing blanks. To get the length without trailing blanks, use LENGTH(RTRIM(strexpr)).

LG10(numexpr) *Numeric* Returns the logarithm with base 10 of numexpr, which must be numeric and greater than 0.

LN(numexpr) *Numeric* Returns the natural logarithm (base e) of numexpr, which must be numeric and greater than 0.

LOWER(strexpr) *String* Returns strexpr with upper-case letters changed to lower case and other characters unchanged.

LPAD(strexpr,length) *String* Returns the string strexpr padded on the left with blanks to extend it to the length given by length, which must be a positive integer between 1 and 255.

LPAD(strexpr,length,char) *String* Identical to LPAD with two arguments, but uses char to pad strexpr on the left. The optional third argument char is a single character within apostrophes, or a string expression that yields a single character.

LTRIM(strexpr) *String* Returns the string strexpr trimmed of any leading blanks.

LTRIM(strexpr,char) *String* Identical to LTRIM with one argument, but trims leading instances of char. The optional second argument char is a single character within apostrophes, or a string expression that yields a single character.

MAX(value,value[,...]) *Numeric or string* Returns the maximum value of its arguments that have valid values. It requires two or more arguments.

MEAN(numexpr,numexpr[,...]) *Numeric* Returns the arithmetic mean of its arguments that have valid values.It requires two or more arguments, which must be numeric.

MIN(value,value[,...]) *Numeric or string* Returns the minimum value of its arguments that have valid values. It requires two or more arguments.

MISSING(variable)) *Logical* Returns 1 or true if variable has a missing value. The argument should be a variable name in the working data file.

MOD(numexpr,modulus) *Numeric* Returns the remainder when numexpr is divided by modulus. Both arguments must be numeric, and the modulus must not be zero.

NCDF.distribution(numexpr, ...) *Numeric* Returns the probability that a random variable with a specified noncentral distribution would be less than numexpr.

NMISS(variable[,...]) *Numeric* Returns a count of the arguments that have missing values. It requires one or more arguments, which should be variable names in the working data file.

NORMAL(stddev) *Numeric* Returns a normally distributed pseudo-random number from a distribution with mean 0 and standard deviation stddev, which must be a positive number. You can repeat the sequence of pseudo-random numbers by setting a Seed in the Preferences dialog box before each sequence.

NUMBER(strexpr,format) *Numeric* Returns the value of the string expression str-expr as a number. The second argument, format, is the numeric format used to read strexpr. Thus if name is an 8-character string containing the character representation of a number, NUMBER(name, f8) is the numeric representation of that number. If the string cannot be read using the format, this function returns system-missing.

NVALID(variable[,...]) *Numeric* Returns a count of the arguments that have valid, non-missing values.It requires one or more arguments, which should be variable names in the working data file.

PROBIT(prob) *Numeric* Returns the value in a standard normal distribution with a cumulative probability equal to prob. The argument prob is a probability greater than 0 and less than 1.

RANGE(test,lo,hi[,lo,hi,...]) *Logical* Returns 1 or true if test is within any of the inclusive range(s) defined by the pairs lo, hi. Arguments must be all numeric or all strings of the same length, and each of the lo, hi pairs must be ordered with lo <= hi.

RINDEX(haystack,needle) *Numeric* Returns an integer that indicates the starting position of the last occurrence of the string needle in the string haystack. Returns 0 if needle does not occur within haystack.

RINDEX(haystack,needle,divisor) *Numeric* See the preceding function. The optional third argument divisor is the number of characters used to divide needle into separate strings to be sought. It must be an integer that divides evenly into the length of needle.

RND(numexpr) *Numeric* Returns the integer that results from rounding numexpr, which must be numeric. Numbers ending in .5 exactly are rounded away from zero.

RPAD(strexpr,length) *String* Returns the string strexpr padded on the right with blanks to extend it to the length given by length, which must be a positive integer between 1 and 255.

RPAD(strexpr,length,char) *String* Identical to RPAD with two arguments, but uses char to pad strexpr on the right. The optional third argument char is a single character within apostrophes, or an expression that yields a single character.

RTRIM(strexpr) *String* Returns the string strexpr trimmed of any trailing blanks. This function is normally used within a larger expression, since strings are padded with trailing blanks upon being assigned to variables.

RTRIM(strexpr,char) *String* Identical to RTRIM with one argument, but trims trailing instances of char. The optional second argument char is a single character within apostrophes, or an expression that yields a single character.

RV.distribution(prob, ...) *Numeric* Returns a random number sampled from a specified distribution.

SD(numexpr,numexpr[,...]) *Numeric* Returns the standard deviation of its arguments that have valid values. It requires at least two arguments, which must be numeric.

SIN(radians) *Numeric* Returns the sine of a numeric value measured in radians.

SQRT(numexpr) *Numeric* Returns the positive square root of numexpr, which must be numeric and not negative.

STRING(numexpr,format) *String* Returns the string that results when numexpr is converted to a string according to format. STRING(-1.5,F5.2) returns the string value '-1.50'. The second argument format must be a format for writing a numeric value.

SUBSTR(strexpr,pos) *String* Returns the substring beginning at position pos of strexpr and running to the end of strexpr.

SUBSTR(strexpr,pos,length) *String* Returns the substring beginning at position pos of strexpr and running for length length.

SUM(numexpr,numexpr[,...]) *Numeric* Returns the sum of its arguments that have valid values. It requires two or more arguments, which must be numeric.

SYSMIS(numvar)) *Logical* Returns 1 or true if the value of numvar is system-missing. The argument numvar must be the name of a numeric variable in the working data file.

TIME.DAYS(days) *Numeric in SPSS time-interval format* Returns a time interval corresponding to the indicated number of days. To display this value correctly, assign it a TIME format. The argument must be numeric.

TIME.HMS(hours,min,sec) *Numeric in SPSS time-interval format* Returns a time interval corresponding to the indicated number of hours, min, and sec. To display this value correctly, assign it a TIME format. The arguments must be integers no greater than 24, 60, and 60, respectively, except that the first nonzero argument can exceed its limit, and the last argument can have a fractional part.

TRUNC(numexpr) *Numeric* Returns the value of numexpr truncated to an integer (toward zero).

UNIFORM(max) *Numeric* Returns a uniformly distributed pseudo-random number between 0 and the argument max, which must be numeric (but can be negative). You can repeat the sequence of pseudo-random numbers by setting the same Random Number Seed before each sequence.

UPCAS(strexpr) *String* Returns strexpr with lower-case letters changed to upper case and other characters unchanged.

VALUE(variable) *Numeric or string* Returns the value of variable, ignoring user missing-value definitions for variable, which must be a variable name in the working data file.

VARIANCE(numexpr,numexpr[,...]) *Numeric* Returns the variance of its arguments that have valid values. It requires at least two arguments, which must be numeric.

XDATE.DATE(datevalue) *Numeric in SPSS date format* Returns the date portion from a numeric value in SPSS date format.

XDATE.HOUR(datevalue) *Numeric* Returns the hour (an integer between 0 and 23) from a numeric value in SPSS date format.

XDATE.JDAY(datevalue) *Numeric* Returns the day of the year (an integer between 1 and 366) from a numeric value in SPSS date format.

XDATE.MDAY(datevalue) *Numeric* Returns the day of the month (an integer between 1 and 31) from a numeric value in SPSS date format.

XDATE.MINUTE(datevalue) *Numeric* Returns the minute (an integer between 0 and 59) from a numeric value in SPSS date format.

XDATE.MONTH(datevalue) *Numeric* Returns the month (an integer between 1 and 12) from a numeric value in SPSS date format.

XDATE.QUARTER(datevalue) *Numeric* Returns the quarter of the year (an integer between 1 and 4) from a numeric value in SPSS date format.

XDATE.SECOND(datevalue) *Numeric* Returns the second (a number between 0 and 60) from a numeric value in SPSS date format.

XDATE.TDAY(timevalue) *Numeric* Returns the number of whole days (as an integer) from a numeric value in SPSS time-interval format.

XDATE.TIME(datevalue) *Numeric in SPSS time-interval format, representing the number of seconds since midnight* Returns the time of day from a numeric value in SPSS date format.

XDATE.WEEK(datevalue) *Numeric* Returns the week number (an integer between 1 and 53) from a numeric value in SPSS date format.

XDATE.WKDAY(datevalue) *Numeric* Returns the day-of-week number (an integer between 1, Sunday, and 7, Saturday) from a numeric value in SPSS date format.

XDATE.YEAR(datevalue) *Numeric* Returns the year (as a four-digit integer) from a numeric value in SPSS date format.

YRMODA(year,month,day) *Numeric* Returns the number of days from October 15, 1582 to the date represented by the arguments year, month, and day, which must be integers that form a valid date since October 15, 1582. Two-digit values of year are prefixed with 19.

INDEX